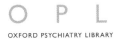

OXFORD PSYCHIATRY LIBRARY

T0177727

Suicide Prevention

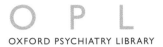

OXFORD PSYCHIATRY LIBRARY

Suicide Prevention

THIRD EDITION

Navneet Kapur

Professor of Psychiatry and Population Health
University of Manchester
United Kingdom

Robert D. Goldney

Emeritus Professor
Discipline of Psychiatry
School of Medicine
University of Adelaide
Australia

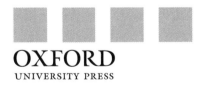

OXFORD
UNIVERSITY PRESS

Great Clarendon Street, Oxford, OX2 6DP,
United Kingdom

Oxford University Press is a department of the University of Oxford.
It furthers the University's objective of excellence in research, scholarship,
and education by publishing worldwide. Oxford is a registered trade mark of
Oxford University Press in the UK and in certain other countries

© Oxford University Press 2019

The moral rights of the authors have been asserted

First Edition published in 2008
Second Edition published in 2013
Third Edition published in 2019

Impression: 1

Published in the United States of America by Oxford University Press
198 Madison Avenue, New York, NY 10016, United States of America

British Library Cataloguing in Publication Data

Data available

Library of Congress Control Number: 2019937234

ISBN 978-0-19-879160-7

Printed in Great Britain by
Bell & Bain Ltd., Glasgow

Foreword

Interest in suicide prevention has never been so high. Public figures talk openly of their suicidal crises, their past self-harm, or the loss of a parent. Claims about the mental health risks of social media make frequent headlines. Many countries worry about young people – are we seeing a more suicidal generation? Bereaved families no longer feel they have to hide their distress, now they demand better support.

With so much more interest, the need to understand the evidence on suicide prevention is also greater than ever. Who are the groups now at highest risk? What are the interventions - from clinic to government department - that could help? What do we mean by risk assessment (clue: it is not prediction)? What have been the benefits of digital, big data and machine learning?

Nav Kapur and Bob Goldney have written a perceptive, comprehensive examination of what we know about suicide prevention, updating the book's excellent predecessors and retaining its clarity of purpose and style. It takes us back to the earliest attempts to understand suicide a couple of centuries ago and tackles the most topical themes in the field - it even has a chapter of rapid fire FAQs. It reflects on the event with the biggest impact on suicide in recent times – the 2008 recession and its aftermath, when an estimated 10,000 "extra" suicides occurred worldwide.

In many areas evidence has improved but remains incomplete. There are too few clinical trials to point to but there are positive findings from other kinds of intervention. Increasingly the most important evidence is international: with 800,000 suicides annually around the world, 75% in low- and middle-income countries, this is a shared problem. The book notes that the largest randomised trial in the whole suicide prevention field was conducted in Sri Lanka.

Some aspects of suicide are deeply troubling. There are parts of the world where suicide is still unlawful. In so many others, stigma and taboo are strong and persistent. But Kapur and Goldney strike a positive tone. People's lives may be complex, risk may be hard to measure, evidence may be patchy, but in the end suicide prevention is possible, and suicide rates in many countries have fallen in recent years. The challenge remains but the book is a convincing account of how it will be met. No suicide, it is telling us, is inevitable.

Louis Appleby MD FRCPsych FRCP
Professor of Psychiatry, University of Manchester
Chair, National Suicide Prevention Strategy Advisory Group,
Dept of Health & Social Care, London.

Preface

Around the turn of the millennium there were a number of multi-author reference books addressing suicidal behaviours. These were comprehensive, detailed, and reflected the many disciplines which could reasonably offer their own perspective. While such volumes were ideal for researchers, they were somewhat daunting for the undergraduate or busy clinician. There appeared to be the need for a concise and evidence-based single-author work, and the first edition of this book evolved. Reassuringly, a second edition was requested, and then a third. By this stage the initial sole contributor had retired, and the next generation of researchers and clinicians had assumed leadership in the field. Professor Nav Kapur therefore joined the writing team and has taken over as primary author for this edition.

Much excellent research has been published since the second edition, and decisions about what to include and leave out were difficult. Of course there will be omissions and gaps, for which the responsibility is ours. What we wanted to end up with was a concise interpretation of the evidence, presented with a practical focus and real-world relevance. We hope readers agree that we have achieved this and that our book contributes in some small way to the prevention of suicide.

Robert (Bob) Goldney, AO, MD, FRCPsych, FRANZCP, Adelaide,
February 2019
Nav Kapur, MBChB, MMedSc, FRCPsych, MD, Manchester,
February 2019

Contents

Acknowledgements

This third edition would not have been completed without the support and love of family and friends. It has been a particular pleasure to be able to share some of the thinking in this book with my children, Priya, Easha, and Rahul.

Our research efforts over the years have been a real team effort. Colleagues, mentors, and patients have all contributed to the ideas in this new edition.

Carol Rayegan-Tafreshi was a great help with administrative support and helping to get the manuscript in shape. Dr Sarah Steeg did brilliant work on the infographics. Dr Alexandra Pitman provided invaluable input on the chapter on bereavement after suicide and Dr Isabelle Hunt kindly provided Figures 5.1 and 11.1. Dr Duleeka Knipe meticulously helped with reference lists, read through the first full draft, and offered insightful comments that helped shape the final version.

I would also like to thank Rachel Goldsworthy, Senior Assistant Commissioning Editor, Oxford University Press for her patience, help, and support, and of course my old friend and mentor, Louis Appleby, for providing a Foreword, as well as his insights over the years. Finally, I would like to thank Bob for this opportunity to work with him. It has been an enormous pleasure and a wonderful learning experience.

NK, Manchester, February 2019

Interaction with patients, clinicians, researchers, and volunteers from many disciplines has been invaluable in refining both my clinical practice and my interpretation of the literature. My long contact with fellow members of the International Association for Suicide Prevention and the International Academy of Suicide Research has also provided valuable insights.

My valued colleague, Professor Johan Schioldann, also contributed to earlier publications which formed the basis for the historical review chapter; and it would be remiss not to acknowledge the support of family members, particularly when one's work/life balance was probably skewed.

Finally, it is a pleasure to acknowledge the overwhelming contribution of Professor Nav Kapur to this third edition. Nav typifies that rare combination of rigorous researcher, caring clinician, and excellent communicator, and I am confident this third edition is stronger for his involvement.

RG, Adelaide, February 2019

Abbreviations

5-HIAA	5-hydroxy indole acetic acid
APA	American Psychiatric Association
BAP	British Association for Psychopharmacology
BMI	body mass index
CATIE	clinical antipsychotic trials of intervention effectiveness
CBT	cognitive behavioural therapy
C-CASA	Columbia Classification Algorithm of Suicide Assessment
CRHT	crisis-resolution home treatment
CSF	cerebrospinal fluid
DBT	dialectical behaviour therapy
DSM	*Diagnostic and Statistical Manual*
DST	dexamethasone suppression test
GABA	gamma-amino butyric acid
HPA	hypothalamic–pituitary–adrenal
IASP	International Association for Suicide Prevention
IASR	International Academy of Suicide Research
IFOTES	International Federation of Telephone Emergency Services
IPT	interpersonal therapy
MCBT	mindfulness-based cognitive behavioural therapy
NICE	National Institute for Health and Care Excellence
NSP	Nordic Consortium on Suicide Prevention
NSSID	non-suicidal self-injury disorder
OSPI Europe	Optimising Suicide Prevention Programs and their Implementation in Europe
PAR	population-attributable risk
PIT	psychodynamic interpersonal therapy
RANZCP	Royal Australian and New Zealand College of Psychiatrists
RCT	randomized controlled trial
SMR	standardized mortality ratio
SPINZ	Suicide Prevention Information New Zealand
SSRI	selective serotonin reuptake inhibitor
TEC	therapeutic evaluative conditioning
WHO	World Health Organization

CHAPTER 1

A brief history of suicidal behaviour

KEY POINTS

- Suicide has been documented since ancient times.
- Systematic research has been conducted for over two hundred years.
- Many of the accepted social and psychiatric antecedents of suicide were well described by the late nineteenth century.

1.1 Historical perspectives and current practice

Although many clinicians and researchers are aware that suicide has been written about since ancient times, in their day-to-day work they tend to ignore publications from previous decades, let alone those from over a hundred years ago. One risk of this is that each generation then needs to rediscover what is important. It would be easy to think that there had not been any suicide research before the German sociologist Emile Durkheim published his classic text *Suicide: A Study in Sociology* (Durkheim, 1897, 1952). In fact, there are well-documented accounts of suicide from antiquity, as well as more detailed inquiries over the last four hundred years (Goldney et al., 2008). Of course, discussion of suicide and the attitudes towards it have varied across time and place. Here we take a largely European historical perspective.

1.2 Suicide in antiquity and the Middle Ages

There are multiple accounts of suicide from ancient Greece and Rome (van Hooff, 1993), and Seidel classified 89 such deaths into categories related to pain and old age, military campaigns, political factors, grief, and mental illness (Seidel, 1995). Some philosophical schools in antiquity had permissive attitudes to suicide—for example the Stoics, who placed great value on reason and control of all aspects of life, including the manner of one's death (Stillion and Stillion, 1999).

Although dying for one's faith was accepted in the early Christian era, attitudes changed over time and suicide came to be regarded as a sin. St Thomas Aquinas argued that suicide was wrong because it was against natural law, it damaged the community, and it did not show respect for the divine gift of life. During this period suicide was deeply stigmatized, with those who died being denied funeral rites and even surviving family members being punished.

1.3 Early English reports

John Sym's *Lifes Preservative Against Self-Killing Or, An Vseful Treatise Concerning Life and Self-Murder* was probably the first book in English to focus exclusively on suicide (Sym, 1637). Sym noted perceptively that 'self-murder is prevented, not so much by arguments against the fact; which disswades from the conclusion; as by the discovery and removall of the motives and causes, whereupon they are tempted to do the same; as diseases are cured by removing of the causes, rather than of their symptoms'.

In 1790 Charles Moore wrote *A Full Inquiry into the Subject of Suicide* (Moore, 1790). He noted 'that there is a sort of madness in "every" act of suicide, even when all idea of lunacy is excluded', and for those who work in the forensic/legal setting and have to determine the state of mind of those who have died by suicide, his comment that 'such distinctions of sanity and insanity are too fine spin to be just or equitable' is particularly pertinent. He also made a number of other observations (see Box 1.1).

Box 1.1 Moore's observations on suicide, 1790

- 'A sort of madness' in all suicide
- Difficulty in distinguishing 'sane and insane suicide'
- Association of alcohol and gambling noted
- Some suicides inherited
- Validity of statistics questioned.

1.4 Nineteenth-century influences

There were significant changes in public attitudes to suicide in the first few decades of the nineteenth century. In England this was associated with the death by suicide, in 1822, of Lord Castlereagh. He had been an influential and successful politician, whose suicide was probably linked to a depressive illness. He was not denied a funeral, as should have been the case, and that led to considerable public debate. This was given further impetus in 1823, when a 22-year-old law student, Abel Griffiths, died by suicide and had the sad misfortune of being the last person to be buried at a crossroads. The rescinding of the law in regard to the treatment of the body of someone who had died by suicide occurred soon after.

The 'medical model' of suicide (suicide essentially being the result of a biologically determined illness) has been attributed primarily to the early nineteenth-century French physician Esquirol, although it is clear that he freely acknowledged the role of social factors as well. A broadly similar approach was offered by Burrows in England, who in 1828 noted that suicide was 'a feature of melancholia', although he added that 'a doubt may naturally arise, whether it be not sometimes perpetrated by a sane mind' (Burrows, 1828). He also referred to the relationship of homicide and infanticide to suicide; the possibility that suicide was 'sometimes innate or hereditary'; that suicide occurred in children; and that contagion could influence suicide. He stated that 'the medical treatment of the propensity to suicide, whether prophylactic or therapeutic, differs not from that which is applicable in cases of ordinary insanity'—a comment still pertinent today.

Social factors were also considered by other early commentators, including Karl Marx, who in 1846 introduced German scholars to the memoirs of Peuchet, the archivist of the Paris Prefecture of Police. In 1838 Peuchet had referred to suicide as a result of 'deficient organisation of our society'. Similarly, the mid-nineteenth-century Norwegian theologian and social researcher Eilert Sundt noted that 'if there is responsibility then it does not only rest on the individual who committed the act, but also on society'.

Significant work occurred in France in the 1850s, including that of Lisle who, in 1856, reviewed over 52,000 suicide deaths, citing 48 causes including insanity, debt, gambling, and 'disappointed love'. Also in 1856, Brierre de Boismont reported on over 4,000 suicide deaths, with no fewer than 18 broad causes. The extent of French contributions to mid-nineteenth-century suicide research can be gauged by noting that bibliographies of the prestigious *Annales Médico-Psychologiques* contain references to 138 papers addressing suicide between 1843 and 1878 (see Box 1.2).

In 1858 Bucknill and Tuke published what was to become the standard textbook of English psychiatry for many years. It contained a classification of three main types of suicide, arising from either suicidal monomania (primary suicidal thoughts and behaviour), melancholia (depression), or delusions and hallucinations (psychosis). There was also a fourth type, defined as instances where it was difficult to determine 'whether the individual was, or was not, a free agent at the time'.

In the United States in the nineteenth century there were research reports and commentaries on suicide, including those in the *American Journal of Insanity*, the forerunner to the *American Journal of Psychiatry*. In the third issue in 1845, the editor, Brigham, commented on the probable under-reporting of suicide deaths, and he also made the following observation on media publicity: 'That suicides are alarmingly frequent in this country is evident to all—and as a means of prevention, we respectfully suggest the propriety of not publishing the details of such occurrences.'

Box 1.2 Mid-nineteenth-century European knowledge

- Importance of insanity in general noted
- Depression (melancholia) and alcohol specifically referred to
- Influence of societal organization discussed
- Interpersonal issues such as 'disappointed love' and 'reversal of fortune' noted
- First classifications of suicide emerged.

1.5 Morselli and late nineteenth-century research

The Italian Morselli published his book *Suicide: An Essay on Comparative Moral Statistics* in 1879, and by 1881 it had been translated into English and German (Morselli, 1879, 1881). It is encyclopaedic in content, and arguably the most important work of nineteenth-century suicidology. Westcott referred to it as a 'thoroughly scientific statistical work', although he added that it was 'hardly a readable book, consisting almost entirely of statistics' (Westcott, 1885); and Tuke referred to it as a 'laborious work for a mass of information' (Tuke, 1892). It contains detailed statistics, focusing on Italy but also including data from a number of other countries. Individual sections of the book included 'Increase and regularity of suicide in civilised countries', 'Social influences', 'Influences arising out of the biological and social conditions of the individual', 'Individual psychological influences', and 'Methods and places of suicide', before Morselli provided a 'Synthesis' on the 'Nature and therapeutics of suicide'.

Morselli analysed age and suicide in different countries, education and suicide rates, and the 'relation of madness with suicide', with the latter demonstrating an association between the numbers of people suffering from 'insanity' and numbers of suicide deaths. He also provided a perceptive view of emotional or psychic pain, noting that 'it is a gross tautological sophism to give the title of "moral suffering" to sorrow for a misfortune, to misery, privation, crossed love or jealousy, whilst they reserve the title of "physical suffering" to pain which arises from a mechanical injury, from an irritation of the peripheral nerves, or disease of the intestines. The cause is unequal, but the effect is the same . . . the expression of moral suffering is the same as that of physical suffering.'

A less statistically focused work than that of Morselli was provided by Westcott, in 1885, in his book *Suicide: Its History, Literature, Jurisprudence, Causation and Prevention*. He addressed the rates and means of suicide—its causes, the effect of urban and rural life, influence of mental disease, suicide from imitation, and effects of physical illness and hereditary factors. He even included a chapter on suicide in animals. This is a surprisingly contemporary set of observations in view of recent ethological conceptualizations of suicide.

Westcott was well aware of the importance of social issues, as in his preface he wrote: 'The question (of suicide) is one well worthy of the earnest consideration of the community; indeed, it may be legitimately regarded as one of our Social Problems, as it involves matters which are intimately connected with our social organization, and is with propriety embraced in our legislative enactments.' It is also of interest, bearing in mind the concerns of some contemporary clinicians, that he observed 'now that a study of suicide as a fact has been instituted, it has fallen almost entirely into a statistical groove, to the neglect of research into the mental state and emotions of the unfortunate individuals who become victims'.

In 1892 there were comprehensive reviews of suicide research by Tuke and Savage in Tuke's *Dictionary of Psychological Medicine* (Tuke, 1892). Tuke presented an erudite historical perspective of suicide, noting that 'there has been no period in authentic history in which, so far as we know, there has been immunity from the practice of self-destruction'. He referred to biblical suicides, then to Greek and Roman perspectives, before noting how attitudes gradually changed over the centuries. His epidemiological review was predominantly of European countries, although data from the United States and Australia were also presented.

Tuke had a critical appreciation of the limitations of some previous research. This is well illustrated in relation to those theories about areas with a high suicide rate and claims that suicide rates were related to geological formations or the weather. Thus, Tuke stated that 'we confess that we accept the conclusions with considerable reserve, first, because the returns of suicide in different countries may differ in their completeness, and therefore may be misleading; and secondly, because the elements of the problem are so exceedingly complex that we are in great danger of referring a maximum amount of suicide to the wrong cause.' Such comments are no less pertinent today than when written by Tuke over a hundred years ago.

Many of Tuke's other observations have stood the test of time and subsequent research: the male to female preponderance of suicide is virtually identical to that found today; it is still the case that 'there is no doubt that agricultural distress increases the number of suicides'; similarly, 'it would seem that divorce exercises a more injurious influence on the male than on the female sex'; suicide remains a reality in children; it is still true that 'the influence of imprisonment on the tendency to suicide . . . (is) well marked, especially in prisoners under 30 years of age', as is the fact that 'the influence of alcohol or beer in the production of suicide is not disputed'; and it is also recognized that 'examples of hereditary suicide have occurred' (see Box 1.3).

Savage provided what could be interpreted as a fairly modern view of mental illness and suicide. He acknowledged that suicide could occur with 'no other signs of insanity', and he also noted that 'in some cases of slight emotional disorder there may be an intention to pretend to commit suicide.' Putting aside the histrocal language, which today would be seen as stigmatizing, this formulation ante-dated the recognition that suicidal behaviour could have a communicative function by 70 years. He also observed that self-mutilation was sometimes

---

Box 1.3 Contemporary relevance of late nineteenth-century research

- Male to female ratio similar
- Importance of depression
- Alcohol influence
- Suicide occurs in children
- Role of contagion noted
- Effect of divorce, rural distress, and prison
- Role of inherited factors acknowledged
- Communication component described
- Noted that self-mutilation provided relief
- Tension between statistical research as opposed to focusing on the individual
- Risk/benefit of different approaches to management discussed.

intended to give relief; that 'all melancholic patients must be considered suicidal till they are fully known'; that even 'simple melancholia of very slight depth is a very common cause of suicide'; and that 'waves of depression occur in many neurotic but otherwise sane people, which often lead to suicide'. He also stated that 'voices may command' and that 'misery produced by constant occurrence of hallucinations, may act like constant pain'.

Savage wrote perceptively that in clinical management 'some risk must be run sooner or later, and it is necessary in curable cases to recognize that the too constant presentation of the idea of distrust to the patient's mind keeps up the morbidly suicidal state', an excellent description of the dilemma facing clinicians treating those who are suicidal.

Savage's work is also notable for his categorization of suicide. He observed that suicide could be either impulsive or deliberate, and the deliberate suicide deaths included those with 'egotistical' and 'altruistic feelings' (see Box 1.4). In fact, these terms had also been documented elsewhere as early as 1880 (Whitt, 2006), albeit without any subsequent attribution by Durkheim who, in 1897, described egoistic, altruistic, anomic, and fatalistic suicide, with the focus being on the predominance of societal influences on suicide (Durkheim, 1897, 1952).

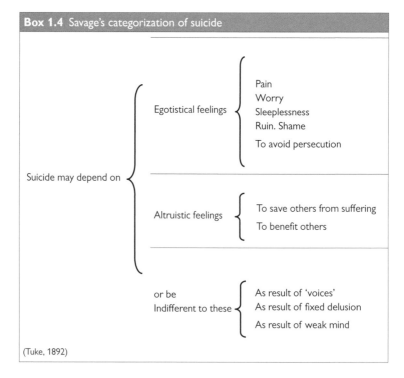

Box 1.4 Savage's categorization of suicide

Suicide may depend on

Egotistical feelings
- Pain
- Worry
- Sleeplessness
- Ruin. Shame
- To avoid persecution

Altruistic feelings
- To save others from suffering
- To benefit others

or be Indifferent to these
- As result of 'voices'
- As result of fixed delusion
- As result of weak mind

(Tuke, 1892)

CHAPTER 1

1.6 Conclusion

This historical review illustrates the breadth and depth of enquiry about suicide that existed prior to the twentieth century (see Figure 1.1 for an overview). Attitudes to suicide varied across the ancient world. In the Middle Ages, the predominant view of suicide, influenced by theological teaching, was that it was sinful. This in time gave way to the more contemporary view of suicide being a result of suffering and something that warranted individual and societal intervention. Suicide came to be viewed as influenced not only by broad social issues, but also by factors such as mental disorders, the media, and occupation, and even hereditary predisposition. Some argued that the reliance on scientific enquiry and empirical data had gone too far, as illustrated by Westcott's comment in 1885 that suicide research had 'fallen almost entirely into a statistical groove'. That suggests that the ground was fertile for the subsequent sociological views of Durkheim and the emerging influence of psychoanalysis, both of which provided a counterpoint to much of the earlier work.

It is clear that in suicidal behaviour research, as in other things, 'new' ideas and paradigms have often been discussed by previous generations. This means that many of the findings of early researchers remain relevant today.

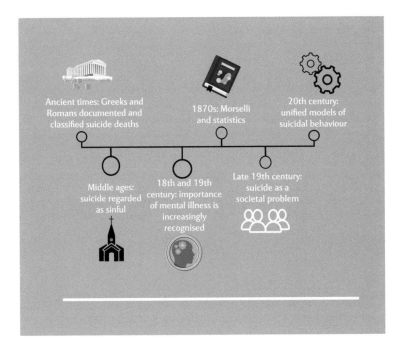

Fig 1.1 A brief history of suicidal behaviour.
Courtesy of Dr Sarah Steeg.

REFERENCES

Brigham, A. (1845). Note by the editor of the *Journal of Insanity*. *American Journal of Insanity* **1**(3): 232–4.

Burrows, G. M. (1828). *Commentaries on the Causes, Forms, Symptoms, and Treatment, Moral and Medical, of Insanity*. London: Thomas and George Underwood.

Durkheim, E. (1897, 1952). *Suicide. A Study in Sociology*. London: Routledge and Kegan Paul.

Goldney, R. D., Schioldann, J. A., and Dunn, K. I. (2008). Suicide research before Durkheim. *Health History* **10**(2): 73–93.

Moore, C. (1790). *A Full Inquiry into the Subject of Suicide etc.* London: J. F. & C. Rivington.

Morselli, E. (1879). *Il Suicidio. Saggio di Statistica Morale Comparata*. Vol. 21 of the *Biblioteca Scientifica Internazionale*. Milano: Dumolard.

Morselli, E. (1881). *Suicide. An Essay on Comparative Moral Statistics*. Revised and abridged by the author for the English version. London: C. Kegan Paul.

Seidel, G. (1995). Suicide in the elderly in antiquity. *International Journal of Geriatric Psychiatry* **10**(12): 1077–84.

Stillion, J. M. and Stillion, B. D. (1999). Attitudes toward suicide: past, present and future. *OMEGA—Journal of Death and Dying* **38**(2): 77–97.

Sym, J. (1637). *Lifes Preservative Against Self-Killing*. London: Dawlman & Fawne.

Tuke, D. H. (1892). *A Dictionary of Psychological Medicine*. London: J. & A. Churchill.

van Hooff, A. J. (1993). Suicide and parasuicide in ancient personal testimonies. *Crisis* **14**(2): 76–82.

Westcott, W. W. (1885). *A Social Science Treatise. Suicide, Its History, Literature, Jurisprudence, Causation and Prevention*. London: H. K. Lewis.

Whitt, H. P. (2006). Durkheim's precedence in the use of the terms egoistic and altruistic suicide: an addendum. *Suicide and Life-Threatening Behavior* **36**(1): 125–7.

CHAPTER 2

Definitions

> **KEY POINTS**
>
> - There are no universally agreed definitions of suicidal behaviour.
> - A variety of terms have been used to try and capture its diversity.
> - A simple pragmatic approach might be most useful because this allows for flexible individualized clinical management.

2.1 Early classification

For well over a hundred years the nomenclature and classification of suicidal behaviour has been controversial. Forty years ago the World Health Organization (WHO) categorized theorists of suicidal behaviour into the Unitarians, for those who saw each attempt as an expression of wishing to die; the Binarians, who saw two groups—those who wished to die by their action and those who had not intended to die; the Pluralists, who saw various intentions in each attempt; and the Individualists, who saw each attempt as a unique episode (Brooke, 1974).

In general, death by suicide may be somewhat easier to classify than non-fatal behaviours. A variety of terms seeking to categorize suicidal behaviours have been used over the years including 'gestures', ambivalent and serious attempts, and intentioned, subintentioned, or unintentioned episodes (Henderson et al., 1977). Attempted suicide has been referred to in a number of ways including pseudocide, parasuicide, acute poisoning, self-injury, and deliberate self-harm (Goldney, 1980; Shneidman, 1985).

2.2 Recent reviews

Reviews have used a plethora of terms for aspects of suicidality, and one paper described nine synonyms for suicidal ideation, nine for suicidal intent, ten for suicide threat or gesture, thirty-six for suicide attempt, and even twenty-seven for suicide itself. Such industry in defining individual behaviour has been reflected in classifications of increasing complexity, resulting in matrices with as many as twenty-seven different categories (Silverman et al., 2007).

A further attempt at categorization was the Columbia Classification Algorithm of Suicide Assessment (C-CASA), which was developed to investigate potential adverse outcomes from antidepressants (Posner et al., 2011). Intrinsic to this classification is the notion that suicidal intent can be reliably delineated. It is arguable whether these developments are of any practical use, although they may be of value from the research point of view. For the clinician, what appears to be of most importance is to determine what the antecedents of the suicidal behaviour may have been, no matter how it is defined.

It is apparent that many of the synonyms and categories refer to several different concepts, often combined. Some refer purely to the semantics of attempted suicide and others to clinical dimensions of suicidal intent and physical lethality.

2.3 The problem with dichotomies

Should people who self-harm be categorized into those who have clear suicidal intent and those who do not? Proponents have argued that a diagnosis of 'non-suicidal self-injury disorder' (NSSID) would increase precision and lead to improved communication between health professionals, as well as stimulate research into causes and prevention, and the development of specific treatments. Others have responded that the term is not useful because suicidal and non-suicidal motivations often co-exist, methods of self-harm change, there is no clear dichotomy of intent in self-harm populations, and even people with low-intent episodes are at increased risk of subsequent suicide (Kapur et al, 2013). It has been suggested that there are potential problems with creating a new diagnosis of NSSID for which there are few proven treatments and which could stigmatize large numbers of young people unnecessarily.

However, the diagnoses of NSSID and attempted suicide disorder are gaining popularity, especially in the United States. They are included in *DSM-5* as conditions requiring further study. Recent taxometric studies (using statistical procedures designed to determine whether constructs are categorical or dimensional) suggest that suicidal ideation in adolescents and suicidal behaviour more generally may be continuously distributed rather than existing as discrete suicidal and non-suicidal subtypes (Liu et al., 2015; Orlando et al., 2015).

It is possible that the dichotomy of those who die and those who survive may have obscured the mixed motivations of these individuals. The overlapping nature of those who die or survive has been long emphasized. The distinction between them is not as clear-cut as is sometimes portrayed. This is illustrated by the fact that the most powerful predictor of suicide is previous suicidal behaviour, no matter how it is defined. The complexity of this area is illustrated by noting that in one study, single emergency-room visits for an overdose, suicidal ideation, or self-harm were each strongly associated with subsequent suicide (Crandall et al., 2006); another study, using the C-CASA, reported that the 'worst-point' lifetime suicidal ideation predicted suicide attempts, but the Scale for Suicide Ideation failed to do so (Posner et al., 2011). Even so-called non-suicidal self-injury is a strong predictor of future suicidal behaviour (Brent, 2011).

Self-harm is the preferred term in the United Kingdom, the earlier prefix 'deliberate' having been dropped because of concerns that it was judgemental and because the extent to which the behaviour is intentional is not always clear. Self-harm refers to an intentional act of self-poisoning or self-injury, irrespective of motivation.

2.4 An ethological/observational approach

Rather than attempting to introduce an artificial certainty into nomenclatures, it might be better to accept that suicidal behaviours are simply relatively non-specific responses to a wide variety of stimuli and mediators.

This is consistent with an ethological conceptualization of suicidal behaviour, with the communication aspect, the so-called 'cry for help', acting as an innate re-lease mechanism, eliciting care from others (Goldney, 1980, 2000). If the suicidal or care-eliciting behaviour is unhelpfully seen by staff or carers to be manipulative or, in ethological terms, cheating, then rejection or, at the very least, ambivalence may be the response.

There appear to be clinical advantages in adopting an observational or ethological conceptualization of suicidal behaviour. By accepting such acts as examples of rela-tively undifferentiated responses to stress, we take into account the environment, the person, the variability of responses, and the mixed motivations and feelings. Such a formulation more readily allows a non-judgemental approach to the patient, with acceptance of both the communication and possible wish to die components.

2.5 Pragmatic definitions

The debate about the nosology of suicidal behaviour could be pursued indefin-itely without satisfying all. It is simpler and probably more helpful to assume that it involves a spectrum in terms of the individual's suicidal intent or wish to die, and the degree of lethality or physical threat to life. Some researchers and clin-icians talk in terms of a 'suicidal process' that ranges from thoughts, through to self-injurious behaviour, and ultimately death by suicide (van Heeringen, 2001). The term 'suicidality' embraces all of these aspects, and within suicidality there are three broad clinical categories (see Table 2.1):

- *Suicide*: a self-inflicted act resulting in death, albeit with varying suicidal intent
- *Non-fatal suicidal behaviour (attempted suicide and self-harm)*: self-injurious behaviour with varying degrees of suicidal intent and lethality
- *Suicidal ideation*: thoughts of self-injurious behaviour with variable suicidal intent, but no lethality.

Table 2.1 Suicidal intent and lethality associated with definitions of suicidal behaviour

	Suicidal intent	Lethality
Suicide	Variable, usually high	Absolute
Non-fatal suicidal behaviour*	Variable	Variable
Suicidal ideation	Variable	Nil

*includes both attempted suicide and self-harm

2.6 Other self-destructive behaviours

We have made no mention of behaviour such as chronic substance abuse or lack of compliance with treatments for potentially fatal physical illness, or even eating disorders. Whether such persons fall under the broad rubric of engaging in suicidal behaviour is open to debate. If we wished to include them, then the same principles of assessment and management that we discuss will generally apply. Of course, such conditions may also be associated with overt suicidal thinking and behavior.

2.7 Conclusion

Simple terminology (suicide, attempted suicide and self-harm, and suicidal ideation) may not find favour with those who prefer complex classifications to accommodate variable degrees of suicidal intent and lethality in a scientifically rigorous manner. However, these terms are easily understood, they are comparatively unambiguous, have stood the test of time, and importantly, they allow for clinical judgement to be exercised in the individual suicidal person. In this book we will use these pragmatic definitions except when referring to specific studies. Whatever definitions are chosen, language of course needs to be used sensitively. Figure 2.1 is an infographic summarizing the information in this chapter.

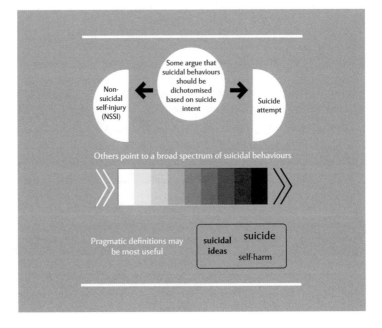

Fig 2.1 Defining suicidal behaviour.
Courtesy of Dr Sarah Steeg.

CHAPTER 2

REFERENCES

Brent, D. (2011). Nonsuicidal self-injury as a predictor of suicidal behavior in depressed adolescents. *Am J Psychiatry* **168**(5): 452–4.

Brooke, E. M. (ed.) (1974). *Suicide and Attempted Suicide*. Public Health Paper No. 58. Geneva: World Health Organization.

Crandall, C., Fullerton-Gleason, L., Aguero, R., and LaValley, J. (2006). Subsequent suicide mortality among emergency department patients seen for suicidal behavior. *Acad Emerg Med* **13**(4): 435–42.

Goldney, R. (2000). Ethology and suicidal behaviour. In *The International Handbook of Suicide and Attempted Suicide,* K. Hawton and K. van Heeringen (eds), pp. 95–106. Chichester: John Wiley.

Goldney, R. D. (1980). Attempted suicide: an ethological perspective. *Suicide Life Threat Behav* **10**(3): 131–41.

Henderson, A. S., Hartigan, J., Davidson, J., et al. (1977). A typology of parasuicide. *Br J Psychiatry* **131**: 631–41.

Kapur, N., Cooper, J., O'Connor, R. C., and Hawton, K. (2013). Non-suicidal self-injury v. attempted suicide: new diagnosis or false dichotomy? *Br J Psychiatry* **202**(5): 326–8.

Liu, R. T., Jones, R. N., and Spirito, A. (2015). Is adolescent suicidal ideation continuous or categorical? A taxometric analysis. *J Abnorm Child Psychol* **43**(8): 1459–66.

Orlando, C. M., Broman-Fulks, J. J., Whitlock, J. L., Curtin, L., and Michael, K. D. (2015). Nonsuicidal self-injury and suicidal self-injury: a taxometric investigation. *Behav Ther* **46**(6): 824–33.

Posner, K., Brown, G. K., Stanley, B., et al. (2011). The Columbia-Suicide Severity Rating Scale: initial validity and internal consistency findings from three multisite studies with adolescents and adults. *Am J Psychiatry* **168**(12): 1266–77.

Shneidman, E. S. (1985). *Definitions of Suicide*. New York: John Wiley.

Silverman, M. M., Berman, A. L., Sanddal, N. D., O'Carroll, W., Joiner, P., and Joiner, T. E. (2007). Rebuilding the tower of Babel: a revised nomenclature for the study of suicide and suicidal behaviors. Part 2: Suicide-related ideations, communications, and behaviors. *Suicide Life Threat Behav* **37**(3): 264–77.

van Heeringen, K. (ed.) (2001). *Understanding Suicidal Behaviour: The Suicidal Process Approach to Research, Treatment and Prevention*. Chichester: Wiley.

CHAPTER 3

Epidemiology

KEY POINTS

- Over 800,000 people die by suicide each year—about three quarters in low- and middle-income countries.
- Twenty to thirty times this number harm themselves.
- Suicide rates globally are under-reported.
- There is wide variation of suicide rates both between and within countries.
- Suicide has increased in middle-aged males in a number of high-income countries.
- Suicidal behaviour and suicidal ideation vary widely in incidence, but they share common antecedents.
- Findings from epidemiological studies do not necessarily apply to the individual person.

3.1 The global burden of suicide

The World Health Organization (WHO) has estimated that around 800,000 people die each year by suicide, representing a global suicide rate of about 11 per 100,000 per year (WHO, 2014). This equates to a suicide death every 40 seconds—a shocking toll. The majority of deaths, perhaps three quarters, occur in low- and middle-income countries. More people die by suicide each year than in wars, and in some countries and age groups (e.g. young people aged 15–29 in high-income countries) more people die by suicide than from motor vehicle accidents. Although overall suicide rates represent an important estimate of the impact, another factor to consider is the effect of premature mortality. Many suicide deaths occur in younger people and measures such as 'potential years of life lost' can help to quantify the societal effect of early death (Gunnell and Middleton, 2003).

3.2 How reliable are the data?

Suicide deaths may be under-reported due to inadequate vital statistics systems, poor quality data, or soceietal stigma. Indeed, suicide remains illegal in some countries (WHO, 2014). Suicide death registration procedures may be complex and conventions for assigning suicide as a cause of death vary. In some countries which rely on legal determination of the cause of death, a 'beyond reasonable doubt' threshold may apply. Criteria can also change over time – in England for example there has been a recent move towards a 'balance of probabilities' judgement. Suicide deaths may sometimes be misclassified as due to accidents or undetermined causes. For this reason in the UK, undetermined deaths tend to be included in national suicide statistics. However, accidental deaths are not.

Despite these challenges, it is generally accepted that official statistics are of value in monitoring changes (Goldney, 2010) but standardized methods of reporting should be pursued (De Leo et al., 2010). Of course, cross-national comparison of suicide rates should be treated with caution. High suicide rates might be considered generally credible but there are exceptions. For example, there was an erroneously high rate of suicide in Sri Lanka based on WHO data which did not reflect recent falls in incidence (Knipe et al., 2015). Very low rates of suicide in some countries may be even more questionable. Rates can be very unstable if a country has a low population and a small number of deaths.

3.3 Suicide rates: an international perspective

The most recently available suicide statistics from a number of different countries are available on the WHO website (http://apps.who.int/gho/data/node.sdg.3-4-data?lang=en). These are based on the WHO global health estimates which use actual mortality data and statistical modelling to estimate rates. These data suggest the highest rates in the Baltic States, Russia, South and Far Eastern Asia, and some countries in East Africa (WHO, 2014). Low rates are reported from some Mediterranean countries and there are even lower rates from elsewhere in the world, but those statistics may be suspect.

Suicide rates vary more than a hundredfold between countries (ranging from 0.4 to 44.2 per 100,000 population). The WHO data suggests that the rate of suicide in high-income countries is slightly higher than in low- and middle-income countries (12.7 versus 11.2 per 100,000 per year), but this could reflect data quality and availability. What is clear is that because the population of low- and middle-income countries is much larger, as many as 75 per cent of all suicide deaths occur in these settings (WHO, 2014). There is also great variation in suicide rates within regions and countries, with a tendency for suicide to be more common in rural than urban areas, as is evident in China and India.

In most countries, suicide is markedly more common in men than women—usually two or three times so. One exception to this in the past had been China, and particularly in rural areas. However, whereas women predominated prior to 2000, since then there has been a reduction in the female suicide rate. This is possibly because of an increase in women's social and economic status in China, and greater geographical mobility, taking women away from potential domestic stressors. The gender gap has narrowed and studies suggest that rates of suicide in China are now higher in men than women in both urban and rural areas (Wang et al., 2014).

Men may have higher rates of suicide worldwide because of their use of more dangerous methods of harm, because of their reluctance to seek help, and because they are more likely to have other risk factors for suicide (e.g. drug and alcohol misuse). Part of the reason for the greater gender parity in the past in rural China, India, and elsewhere may have been due to the high lethality of poisons that were ingested, a method more common in women.

There are marked differences in the incidence of suicide between some ethnic groups, as demonstrated by African Americans having a lower rate of suicide compared with white Americans, although a rise in the suicide rate of African Americans in the 1980s and 1990s has resulted in the rates beginning to converge (Utsey et al., 2007). On the other hand, increased rates in indigenous populations have been reported, including the Canadian Inuit, New Zealand Maori, and Australian Aboriginal People (Lester, 2006). Hispanic Americans and Asian Americans (Duarte-Velez and Bernal, 2007; Leong et al., 2007) also have comparatively high rates of suicide.

In England and Wales, age-standardized suicide rates are lower for South Asian men compared to white males, while women of South Asian origin show slightly elevated rates compared to their white peers (McKenzie et al, 2008).

Factors such as religion, family, and social ties might contribute to the lower suicide rates in some ethnic minority groups (Leong et al., 2007). Factors associated with risk of suicide, such as the stigma of mental health problems, lower rates of contact with mental health services, and substance misuse (Utsey et al., 2007) may contribute to higher suicide rates. The research on ethnic minority groups and suicide is subject to a number of limitations: the selective focus on a small number of ethnic groups; little consideration of the heterogeneity within groups (e.g. the term South Asian in the UK covers people from a variety of countries, cultures, and religions); and limited data (e.g. in England, ethnicity is not routinely recorded on death certificates).

Suicide risk in LGBT communities is a realtively underesearched area but existing studies suggest the incidence of suicidal behavior is elevated (Haas et al.,2011).

3.4 Suicide across the life course

Traditionally, suicide was considered to increase with age, and that remains the case in many countries. In almost all regions worldwide, suicide rates are highest in males and females aged 70 and above (WHO, 2014). However, suicide is also one of the leading causes of death in younger people, accounting for nearly 10 per cent of all deaths in those aged 15–29 years (WHO, 2014).

Since the 1990s there has been a decline in suicide rates among 15 to 24-year-olds (especially males) in many Western countries (Varnik et al., 2009). This may be partly associated with the implementation of national suicide prevention programmes or to treatment-related factors such as increases in antidepressant prescribing (Gibbons et al., 2006). Suicide rates in older adults may also have shown a decline (Shah et al., 2008). As a result of these age-related changes, the age profile of suicide has altered considerably.

Although broadly speaking, suicide rates do increase with advancing age, there are greater numbers of suicide among younger and middle-aged adults in some countries. For example, in the UK in 2015 suicide was most frequent in men aged 40–59 years, followed by men aged 30–44 years (Office for National Statistics, 2017).

3.5 Methods of suicide

There are differences in the methods of suicide among countries (Ajdacic-Gross et al., 2008). Common methods by country include:

- *In England and Wales*: hanging, poisoning with drugs
- *In the USA:* firearms, hanging, and poisoning with drugs
- *In Sweden:* poisoning with drugs, hanging, and firearms
- *In Hungary:* hanging, poisoning with drugs, and jumping from a height
- *In India:* poisoning with pesticides, hanging, and self-immolation
- *In China:* hanging, poisoning with pesticides, drowning
- *In Australia and New Zealand*: hanging, poisoning with drugs.

The important influence of the predominant method of suicide on a country's suicide rate was highlighted by the sustained reduction in suicide in the UK following the introduction of non-toxic North Sea gas into domestic supplies in 1958—the so-called 'coal gas story'. It is also illustrated in those countries where the predominant mode of suicide is agricultural pesticides. It is probable that this very lethal method of suicide is at least in part responsible for the high rates in Asia. This contrasts with the ready availability of less toxic tranquilizers and analgesics being used in Western countries, which means that 'impulsive' overdoses are less likely to lead to death.

3.6 Suicide rates over time

The WHO compared suicide rates among 172 member states between 2000 and 2012. In nearly half (49 per cent) of the countries there had been a drop in suicide rates of over 10 per cent between these time periods; 17 per cent showed an increase of over 10 per cent; and 34 per cent showed changes of between minus 10 per cent and plus 10 per cent (WHO, 2014).

The recent global economic recession of 2008–2010 has generated a number of empirical studies examining its effect on national suicide rates. Chang and colleagues (2013) examined the impact of the economic crisis on suicide rates in 54 European and American countries. They found 4,884 excess suicide deaths in 2009 compared with the expected number based on trends before the crisis. Other studies have reported that this economic crisis has contributed to an estimated 10,000 additional suicide deaths in Europe, Canada, and the USA (Reeves et al., 2014).

The considerable variation of suicide rates over relatively short periods of time—such as the threefold increase in suicide in young males in high-income countries in the latter decades of the twentieth century, or the more recent increase among men in mid life—does not have a simple explanation. The following could all be implicated:

- Limited employment opportunities
- Increasing use of substances, particularly alcohol and street drugs
- Changed gender roles
- Changes in the delivery of healthcare or help seeking behaviour
- A cohort effect—the at-risk cohort of young men from 20 or 30 years ago have simply grown older.

3.7 The 'iceberg model' of suicidal behaviour

It has been suggested that the epidemiology of suicidal behaviour might be best understood as an iceberg (see Figure 3.1). Behaviours become more common, but less severe and less visible, as one descends the iceberg. The most serious episodes are at the top—deaths by suicide. Self-harm which comes to medical attention is the next level of the iceberg. Even when people present to hospitals, some episodes may go unrecognized and are hence 'under the surface'.

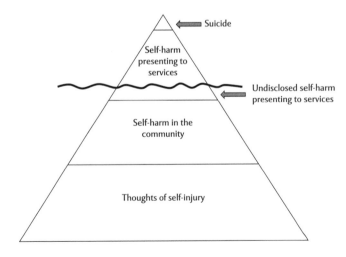

Fig 3.1 The 'iceberg' model of suicidal behaviour.

Self-harm in the community may be hidden and never come to the attention of health or helping services. Below this there may be an even larger group of people who experience thoughts of self-injury without acting on them. The important point to note is that the majority of epidemiological research in self-harm has been carried out in hospital settings. Recently, however, there have been attempts to quantify the different levels of the iceberg (Geulayov et al., 2018).

3.8 Attempted suicide and self-harm

These terms are sometimes used interchangeably. Self-harm is a multifaceted and complex behaviour varying in both severity and intent and includes intentional acts of self-poisoning and self-injury (Kapur, 2009). There are international differences in the nomenclature used, with some distinguishing between 'non-suicidal self-injury' and 'suicide attempt' (see Chapter 2). There is continuing debate about the strength of the evidence upon which such a distinction is based (Kapur et al., 2013). Non-fatal behaviours are much more common than suicide—perhaps around 30 times more common in some settings—but data are often less readily available.

School- and community-based surveys are a useful source of information. In the international Child and Adolescent Self-harm in Europe Study, Madge and colleagues reported rates for self-harm in the previous year of 8.9 per cent for females and 2.6 per cent for males, and lifetime rates of 13.5 per cent and 4.3 per cent respectively (Madge et al., 2008). In a community survey of adults, Nock et al. assessed the prevalence of suicidal ideation, plans, and attempts using the Composite International Diagnostic Interview as part of the WHO World Mental Health Survey initiative (Nock et al., 2008). Across 17 high-, middle-, and low-income countries, the lifetime prevalence of suicide attempts was 2.7 per cent, with a lifetime prevalence of 9.2 per cent for ideation and 3.1 per cent for suicide planning. There was substantial cross-national variability, with the lifetime prevalence of suicide attempts ranging from 0.7 per cent in Nigeria to 5 per cent in the USA.

Other studies have estimated rates of self-harm based on hospital attendances. In England, self-harm data are available from 2000 for the three sites that make up the Multi-Centre Project of Self-harm (Oxford, Manchester, Derby) (http:// cebmh.warne.ox.ac.uk/csr/mcm/). In 2014, the rates of self-harm were 320 per 100,000 per year for men and 445 per 100,000 per year for women. The peak age of presentation during the study period (2000–2014) was 15–24 years for women (42 per cent of female episodes). Men had a more even age distribution, with approximately one third of men who self-harmed aged 15–24 years and one third aged 35–54 years. Self-poisoning featured in 74 per cent of episodes, self-injury (mostly cutting) in 21 per cent, with both self-poisoning and self-injury occurring together in the remainder of episodes.

In many countries there is concern about a possible increase in self-harm among young people. A recent UK study based in primary care reported a specific 70 per cent increase in rates of self-harm in girls aged 13–16 years but no increase in adjacent age groups or in boys (Morgan et al., 2017). Possible explanations are related to increases in psychological distress as a result of contemporary pressures on young girls in this age group. It was also suggested that social media may have played a role.

Suicide and self-harm are separate but overlapping behaviours. However, their antecedents are the same; it may be chance that determines survival or death; and those who self-harm are at least 30 times more likely to die by suicide during the following year than the general population.

In an important review of the worldwide literature, Carroll et al. found that in the year after a self-harm episode, the incidence of suicide was 1.6 per cent and the incidence of repeat self-harm was 16.3 per cent (Carroll et al., 2014). Bergen and colleagues suggested that presenting to hospital with self-harm was associated with a significantly lower life expectancy—between 30 and 40 years of life lost when external causes of death (such as suicide and accidents) were considered (Bergen et al., 2012). In terms of the prognosis for self-harm in young people, there were more positive findings from the study by Moran and colleagues—nine out of ten young people who reported self-harm during adolescence (mean age of the sample 15.9 to 17.4 years) did not go on to self-harm as adults (Moran et al., 2012).

3.9 Suicidal ideation

Suicidal ideation can vary between fleeting thoughts that life is not worth living, to profound firmly held beliefs that suicide is the only answer. This variation is reflected in a broad range of prevalence estimates. Some general population studies have given a figure of about 3–4 per cent of the population having a significant degree of suicidal ideation in any one year (Pirkis et al., 2000). A recent general population psychiatric survey from the UK found that 5.4 per cent of adults aged 16–74 years reported suicidal thoughts in the previous year (McManus et al., 2016). There is overlap between suicidal ideation and other suicidal behaviours. Follow-up studies have shown a strong association with future attempted suicide and death by suicide (Kuo et al., 2001).

3.10 The 'tipping point' and cohort effect

The concept of the 'tipping point' implies that there is a background base rate of a phenomenon resulting from many factors, which when exceeded (for reasons which may not be immediately apparent) results in a dramatic increase in that phenomenon, perhaps through imitation, social learning, or normalizing effects. It may help us to understand changes such as the fluctuations in the rates of suicide and self-harm (Goldney, 1998). It also offers some explanation for the observation of a cohort effect, where people in specific age groups—who have been exposed to broadly similar early life experiences, and developmental and sociological factors—may carry their vulnerability with them throughout life (Snowdon and Hunt, 2002; Gunnell et al., 2003).

3.11 Conclusion

Epidemiological studies provide powerful evidence for the importance of biopsycho-social influences on suicide rates, and they can guide policy makers in identifying and prioritizing suicide prevention initiatives. However, clinicians must be aware of the ecological fallacy of extrapolating from large epidemiological data to an individual person. When assessing someone who is suicidal, a more focused clinical approach is needed. Figure 3.2 is an infographic summarizing the information in this chapter.

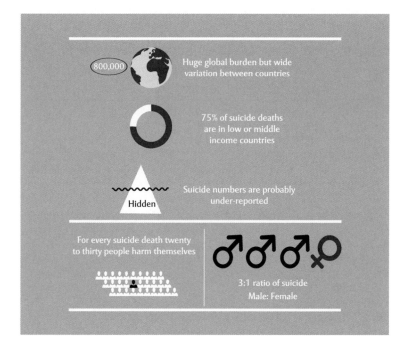

Fig 3.2 The epidemiology of suicidal behaviour.
Courtesy of Dr Sarah Steeg.

REFERENCES

Ajdacic-Gross, V., Weiss, M. G., Ring, M., et al. (2008). Methods of suicide: international suicide patterns derived from the WHO mortality database. *Bull World Health Organ* **86**(9): 726–32.

Bergen, H., Hawton, K., Waters, K., et al. (2012). Premature death after self-harm: a multicentre cohort study. *Lancet* **380**(9853): 1568–74.

Carroll, R., Metcalfe, C., and Gunnell, D. (2014). Hospital presenting self-harm and risk of fatal and non-fatal repetition: systematic review and meta-analysis. *PLoS One* **9**(2): e89944.

De Leo, D., Dudley, M. J., Aebersold, C. J., et al. (2010). Achieving standardised reporting of suicide in Australia: rationale and program for change. *Med J Aust* **192**(8): 452–6.

Duarte-Velez, Y. M. and Bernal, G. (2007). Suicide behavior among Latino and Latina adolescents: conceptual and methodological issues. *Death Stud* **31**(5): 435–55.

Geulayov, G., Casey, D., McDonald, K. C., et al. (2018). Incidence of suicide, hospital-presenting non-fatal self-harm, and community-occurring non-fatal self-harm in adolescents in England (the iceberg model of self-harm): a retrospective study. *Lancet Psychiatry* **5**(2): 167–74.

Gibbons, R. D., Hur, K., Bhaumik, D. K., and Mann, J. J. (2006). The relationship between antidepressant prescription rates and rate of early adolescent suicide. *Am J Psychiatry* **163**(11): 1898–904.

Goldney, R. D. (1998). Variation in suicide rates: the 'tipping point'. *Crisis* **19**(3): 136–8.

Goldney, R. D. (2010). A note on the reliability and validity of suicide statistics. *Psychiatry, Psychol Law* **17**(1): 52–6.

Gunnell, D. and Middleton, N. (2003). National suicide rates as an indicator of the effect of suicide on premature mortality. *The Lancet* **362**(9388): 961–2.

Gunnell, D., Middleton, N., Whitley, E., Dorling, D., and Frankel, S. (2003). Influence of cohort effects on patterns of suicide in England and Wales, 1950–1999. *Br J Psychiatry* **182**: 164–70.

Haas, A. P., Eliason, M., Mays, V. M., et al. Suicide and suicide risk in lesbian, gay, bisexual, and transgender populations: review and recommendations. *J Homosex* 2011; **58**: 10–51.

Kapur, N. (2009). Self-harm in the general hospital. *Psychiatry* **8**(6): 189–93.

Kapur, N., Cooper, J., O'Connor, R. C., and Hawton, K. (2013). Non-suicidal self-injury v. attempted suicide: new diagnosis or false dichotomy? *Br J Psychiatry* **202**(5): 326–8.

Knipe, D. W., Metcalfe, C., and Gunnell, D. (2015). WHO suicide statistics—a cautionary tale. *Ceylon Med J* **60**(1): 35.

Kuo, W. H., Gallo, J. J., and Tien, A. Y. (2001). Incidence of suicide ideation and attempts in adults: the 13-year follow-up of a community sample in Baltimore, Maryland. *Psychol Med* **31**(7): 1181–91.

Leong, F. T., Leach, M. M., Yeh, C., and Chou, E. (2007). Suicide among Asian Americans: what do we know? What do we need to know? *Death Stud* **31**(5): 417–34.

Lester, D. (2006). Suicide among indigenous peoples: a cross-cultural perspective. *Arch Suicide Res* **10**(2): 117–24.

Madge, N., Hewitt, A., Hawton, K., et al. (2008). Deliberate self-harm within an international community sample of young people: comparative findings from the Child & Adolescent Self-harm in Europe (CASE) Study. *J Child Psychol Psychiatry* **49**(6): 667–77.

McKenzie, K., Bhui, K., Nanchahal, K., and Blizard, B. (2008). Suicide rates in people of South Asian origin in England and Wales: 1993–2003. *Br J Psychiatry* **193**(5): 406–9.

McManus, S., Bebbington, P., Jenkins, R., and Brugha, T. (2016). *Mental Health and Wellbeing in England: Adult Psychiatric Morbidity Survey 2014*. Leeds: NHS Digital.

Moran, P., Coffey, C., Romaniuk, H., et al. (2012). The natural history of self-harm from adolescence to young adulthood: a population-based cohort study. *Lancet* **379**(9812): 236–43.

Morgan, C., Webb, R. T., Carr, M. J., et al. (2017). Incidence, clinical management, and mortality risk following self harm among children and adolescents: cohort study in primary care. *BMJ* **359**: j4351.

Nock, M. K., Borges, G., Bromet, E. J., et al. (2008). Cross-national prevalence and risk factors for suicidal ideation, plans and attempts. *Br J Psychiatry* **192**(2): 98–105.

Office for National Statistics (2017). *Suicide Occurrences, England and Wales*. From https:// www.ons.gov.uk/peoplepopulationandcommunity/birthsdeathsandmarriages/deaths/ datasets/suicideinenglandandwales

Pirkis, J., Burgess, P., and Dunt, D. (2000). Suicidal ideation and suicide attempts among Australian adults. *Crisis* **21**(1): 16–25.

Reeves, A., McKee, M., and Stuckler, D. (2014). Economic suicides in the Great Recession in Europe and North America. *Br J Psychiatry* **205**(3): 246–7.

Shah, A., Bhat, R., MacKenzie, S., and Koen, C. (2008). Elderly suicide rates: cross-national comparisons of trends over a 10-year period. *Int Psychogeriatr* **20**(4): 673–86.

Snowdon, J. and Hunt, G. E. (2002). Age, period and cohort effects on suicide rates in Australia, 1919–1999. *Acta Psychiatr Scand* **105**(4): 265–70.

Utsey, S. O., Hook, J. N., and Stanard, P. (2007). A re-examination of cultural factors that mitigate risk and promote resilience in relation to African American suicide: a review of the literature and recommendations for future research. *Death Stud* **31**(5): 399–416.

Varnik, A., Kolves, K., Allik, J., et al. (2009). Gender issues in suicide rates, trends and methods among youths aged 15–24 in 15 European countries. *J Affect Disord* **113**(3): 216–26.

Wang, C. W., Chan, C. L., and Yip, P. S. (2014). Suicide rates in China from 2002 to 2011: an update. *Soc Psychiatry Psychiatr Epidemiol* **49**(6): 929–41.

World Health Organization (2014). *Preventing Suicide: A Global Imperative 2014*. From http://www.who.int/mental_health/suicide-prevention/world_report_2014/en/

CHAPTER 4

What causes suicidal behaviour?

KEY POINTS

- Psychological autopsy studies suggest that as many as 80–90 per cent of people who die by suicide may have a psychiatric illness at the time of death.
- Measures of population impact also highlight the importance of mental disorders.
- However, the causes of suicide are multiple and complex.
- The stress diathesis model is a useful framework to understand suicidal behaviour.
- The presence of even multiple risk factors is not sufficient to explain suicide—an individualized approach is needed when assessing patients.

4.1 Introduction

One of the most common questions professionals are asked after someone harms themselves or dies by suicide is 'why has this happened?' This chapter will discuss some of the possible causes of suicidal behavior, but it is important to remember that suicide is complex. The contributing factors are rarely easily characterized.

4.2 The psychological autopsy approach

Some studies have used a 'psychological autopsy approach' which involves the collection of information about people who have died by suicide, from a variety of clinical and personal sources. Such studies typically involve interviews with family members, relatives, friends, and healthcare staff. This allows detailed collection of relevant information but, because of the retrospective nature of the investigation, the findings may be subject to recall bias (Hawton et al., 1998). Work from a number of countries has suggested that as many as 80–90 per cent of those who die by suicide may have mental disorders, particularly depression, at the time of their death. It has also been argued that most of those persons without a diagnosis at the time of death probably had an underlying psychiatric condition that was not detected by the psychological autopsy method (Ernst et al., 2004).

However, such findings may not be universally applicable, as less mental disorder has been found in those who die by suicide in China, India, and possibly other low- and middle-income countries. This may be due to high-lethality methods (e.g. poisoning by agrochemicals) being used in those countries, whereas in higher-income countries less toxic medications are taken in overdose (Phillips,

2010). The lower prevalence of psychiatric disorder might also reflect the very different sociocultural context. This is an important illustration of the need to be cautious before we try to generalize our understanding of suicidal behaviour.

4.3 Other research methodologies

Other research techniques have included:

- twin studies, which can help delineate the relative importance of inherited as well as environmental factors. Such research suggests that the heritable proportion of suicidal behaviour is between 30 and 50 per cent (Voracek and Loibl, 2007).

case-control studies of those who attempt suicide, which have emphasized the importance of mood disorders and substance abuse (Beautrais et al., 1996)

large retrospective cohort studies, which have demonstrated a graded relationship to attempted suicide of adverse childhood experiences including emotional, physical, and sexual abuse, substance abuse, mental illness, incarceration, and parental domestic violence, separation, or divorce (Dube et al., 2001).

- longitudinal cohort analyses, which have shown that suicidal behaviour is strongly associated with prior suicidal behaviour and self-harm (Bergen et al., 2012) and influenced by an accumulation of factors including family history of suicide, childhood sexual abuse, personality factors, peer contacts, and school success or failure (Fergusson et al., 2003). Danish register research has demonstrated an increasing gradation of suicide risk for those who had mild, moderate, or severe depression, confirming clinical beliefs about the prognosis and suicide risk of those with increasing degrees of depression (Kessing, 2004).

4.4 Factors associated with suicide

Many different factors contribute to suicide risk (see Box 4.1). Some authors refer to risk factors as distal (longstanding or trait variables) or proximal (acute or state variables) (Hawton and van Heeringen, 2009). Risk factors range from genetic, to neurodevelopmental factors, to childhood and later experiences, as well as psychological and clinical factors. Whole communities may be at increased risk (e.g. those from LGBT groups) and suicide may be more common in ceratin occupations (e.g. lower skilled jobs, construction workers or individuals with increased access to lethal means of suicide such as health professionals). It is evident that many of these risk factors, particularly those in childhood and adolescence, are not specific to suicidal behaviours, as they are related to mental disorders in general. Some factors are modifiable (e.g. depression), but others are not (e.g. age).

Box 4.1 Risk factors for suicide

Distal

- Genetic loading
- Personality characteristics (e.g. impulsivity, aggression)
- Restricted fetal growth and perinatal circumstances
- Early traumatic life events
- Neurobiological disturbances (e.g. serotonin dysfunction and hypothalamic-pituitary axis hyperactivity)

Proximal

- Psychiatric disorder
- Physical disorder
- Psychosocial crisis
- Availability of means
- Exposure to models or people who have died

Adapted from *The Lancet*, 373, Hawton K., van Heeringen K., Suicide, pp. 1372-1381. Copyright (2009) with permission from Elsevier. DOI:https://doi.org/10.1016/S0140-6736(09)60372-X

It is also important to appreciate that not all risk factors are of equal importance. Some characteristics may greatly increase risk; others may increase risk only moderately but be particularly common in the population as a whole.

Research has also pointed to the importance of the recognition and adequate treatment of mental disorders as possible protective factors. The lack of consistency between the use of psychotropic medication at the time of suicide and the patterns of diagnoses made at psychological autopsy has been noted (Marzuk et al., 1995); there is often a lack of continuity of care (Hulten and Wasserman, 1998); there is frequently an absence of enquiry about suicidal thoughts, particularly in the elderly (Waern et al., 1999); and there is often a reduction in the intensity of care prior to suicide (The National Confidential Inquiry into Suicide and Homicide by People with Mental Illness, 2001).

4.5 Relative importance of contributing factors

Some of the Danish register studies have been particularly valuable in investigating the relative importance of different risk factors, as they have used the population attributable risk (PAR) statistic. The PAR is a measure of the proportion of a condition that may be associated with exposure to a risk factor, or the proportion of the condition that would be eliminated if the risk factor was not present (assuming a causal relationship). The PAR is helpful for assessing the differing impact of various contributing factors to suicidal behaviour, as it allows risk factors at the population level to be placed in perspective. It can be illustrated by considering the association between smoking and lung cancer. It is accepted that smoking causes lung cancer, but not in everyone who smokes. The PAR of smoking for lung cancer is about 80 per cent (Siegel et al., 2015), which means that if all smoking were eliminated, approximately 80 per cent of all lung cancer cases would be prevented. Similarly, the various PARs for factors related to suicidal behaviour can be calculated, although the causal relationships may be less well established.

In a Danish register examination of data for 21,169 people who had died by suicide and 423,128 controls, the PAR for suicide of ever having had a mental disorder necessitating hospital admission was 40.3 per cent, whereas those PARs for suicide of other factors, including unemployment, having a sickness-related absence from work, being in the lowest-income quartile, and being on a disability or age pension were 2.8 per cent, 6.4 per cent, 8.8 per cent, 3.2 per cent, and 10.2 per cent, respectively (Qin et al., 2003). While these other issues cannot be ignored, the study suggests that one focus of attention might be on those persons who have required hospitalization for mental disorders.

The PAR statistic has been used by other researchers with broadly similar re-sults. For example, there have been a number of studies demonstrating that de-pression has a PAR of approximately 40 per cent for suicide, attempted suicide, and even suicidal ideation, and there is an even greater PAR for depression in suicide in older adults (Beautrais, 2002; Goldney et al., 2003). In a large system-atic review, the population-attributable fraction for mental disorder overall was calculated to range from 40 to 70 per cent (Cavanagh et al., 2003).

When considering repeat suicidal behaviour (rather than death by suicide) as an outcome, a large English study reported that the PAR of a past history of suicidal behaviour was over 40 per cent (Kapur et al., 2006).

It is important to note that these PAR results are valid only for the populations studied, that is, in high-income countries with well-developed health and social services, and they would not necessarily be applicable to low- and middle-income countries. Psychiatric disorder and previous suicidal behaviour are probably the most important risk factors for suicide in high-income countries, but others cannot be ignored. The role of psychosocial and societal influences on suicidal behaviour is discussed in later chapters. Of course another caveat with the PAR is that not all associations at a population level will be causal and not all risk factors will be modifiable.

Physical illness can also be an important contributing factor, particularly in older adults. Renal haemodialysis and transplantation, neoplasms (particularly those of the head and neck), AIDS/HIV, systemic lupus, and spinal cord injuries have all been associated with increased rates of suicide (Stenager and Stenager, 2000). A large primary care based study from the UK suggested that the rate of sui-cide was significantly elevated in people with a range of physical illnesses, es-pecially in women. The presence of depression largely explained the elevated risks, although not in women with cancer or coronary heart disease (Webb et al., 2012). Even in the other groups, it is possible that the physical illness resulted in depression which then led to suicide—so depression was on the causal pathway rather than being a confounder. Another study found that risks were elevated when the physical and psychiatric illnesses occurred close in time to one another. The exact sequence was less important (Qin et al., 2014).

4.6 Drawing risk factors together—models of suicidal behaviour

Although risk factors may provide some clues to aetiology, they are unable to explain why suicide and self-harm occur. Explanatory models may help us to understand the phenomena better, help to formulate testable hypotheses, and ultimately facilitate the development of appropriate treatments. One of the most influential models of suicidal behaviour is a clinical model—the stress diathesis or stress vulnerability model. This suggests that certain individuals carry with them a predisposition to suicidal behaviour (which may be related to sex, religion, familial and genetic factors, childhood experiences, psychosocial support systems, access to lethal methods, or biological factors). The vulnerability only leads to suicidal behaviour when the individual encounters a stressor (which could be a mental

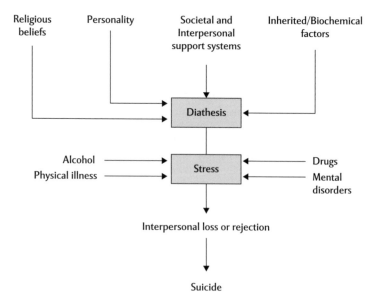

Fig 4.1 The stress diathesis model of suicidal behaviour.

disorder, alcohol or drug misuse, a medical illness, or a psychosocial crisis). The model is summarized in Figure 4.1.

Other influential models of suicidal behaviour include the 'Cry of Pain' model (which emphasizes the role of defeat and entrapment—the sense there is no-where else to go following the experience of a major stressor), the Interpersonal-Psychological model (which suggests perceived burdensomeness and thwarted belongingness are central to suicidal ideation), and the Integrated Motivational-Volitional model—a stress diathesis model which highlights the pre-motivational, motivational (ideation and intent formation), and volitional (behavioural, en-action) phases of suicidality. A full review is provided in O'Connor and Nock (2014).

4.7 The Haddon Matrix

While the stress/diathesis conceptualization of suicidal behaviour is probably the most accepted in clinical practice, another model that might allow a clearer delineation of the 'where, how, and who' of suicide prevention is the Haddon Matrix (Eddleston et al., 2006). This is a public health injury prevention model, based on the host or individual person, the agent or means of suicidal behaviour, and the environment (including the person's personal and community relationships). The components of the model as applied to suicidal behaviour are summarized in Table 4.1.

Table 4.1 Haddon Matrix of factors influencing suicidal behaviour and its outcomes			
	Individual	Means of suicidal behaviour	Environment
Pre-suicidal factors	Age Gender Personality Mental disorders Substance abuse Inherited factors Physical illness	Accessibility of: drugs, firearms, pesticides, jumping sites	Personal relationships Community support Media influences
Suicidal behaviour	Substance intoxication Interpersonal rejection Suicidal intent	Lethality of method	Proximity to others Likelihood of discovery/ prevention
Post-suicidal factors	Help-seeking General health Compliance with treatment	Effectiveness of acute and follow-up treatment	Availability of treatment Social and personal support network

4.8 Conclusion

Large-scale research has demonstrated conclusively the importance of psychiatric illness, previous suicidal behaviour, psychosocial factors, and physical illnesses. However, none of those factors is sufficient to fully explain suicidal behaviour on an individual level. Even with an accumulation of such factors, a person's perception of his or her environment, interpersonal stressors, and relationships are still of critical importance. Some people with many risk factors have no history of suicidal behaviour, and others with few risk factors may still die by suicide. This highlights the complexity of the issue and the importance of an individualized approach to assessment. We explore this further in Chapter 7. Figure 4.2 is an infographic summarizing the information in this chapter.

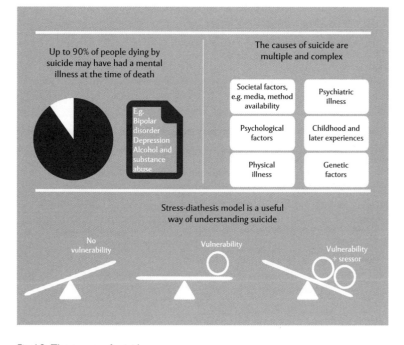

Fig 4.2 The causes of suicide.
Courtesy of Dr Sarah Steeg.

REFERENCES

Beautrais, A. L. (2002). A case control study of suicide and attempted suicide in older adults. *Suicide Life Threat Behav* **32**(1): 1–9.

Beautrais, A. L., Joyce, P. R., Mulder, R. T., Fergusson, D. M., Deavoll, B. J., and Nightingale, S. K. (1996). Prevalence and comorbidity of mental disorders in persons making serious suicide attempts: a case-control study. *Am J Psychiatry* **153**(8): 1009–14.

Bergen, H., Hawton, K., Waters, K., et al. (2012). Premature death after self-harm: a multicentre cohort study. *Lancet* **380**(9853): 1568–74.

Cavanagh, J. T., Carson, A. J., Sharpe, M., and Lawrie, S. M. (2003). Psychological autopsy studies of suicide: a systematic review. *Psychol Med* **33**(3): 395–405.

Dube, S. R., Anda, R. F., Felitti, V. J., Chapman, D. P., Williamson, D. F., and Giles, W. H. (2001). Childhood abuse, household dysfunction, and the risk of attempted suicide throughout the life span: findings from the Adverse Childhood Experiences Study. *JAMA* **286**(24): 3089–96.

Eddleston, M., Buckley, N. A., Gunnell, D., Dawson, A. H., and Konradsen, F. (2006). Identification of strategies to prevent death after pesticide self-poisoning using a Haddon matrix. *Inj Prev* **12**(5): 333–7.

Ernst, C., Lalovic, A., Lesage, A., Seguin, M., Tousignant, M., and Turecki, G. (2004). Suicide and no axis I psychopathology. *BMC Psychiatry* **4**: 7.

Fergusson, D. M., Beautrais, A. L., and Horwood, L. J. (2003). Vulnerability and resiliency to suicidal behaviours in young people. *Psychol Med* **33**(1): 61–73.

Goldney, R. D., Dal Grande, E., Fisher, L. J., and Wilson, D. (2003). Population attributable risk of major depression for suicidal ideation in a random and representative community sample. *J Affect Disord* **74**(3): 267–72.

Hawton, K., Appleby, L., Platt, S., et al. (1998). The psychological autopsy approach to studying suicide: a review of methodological issues. *J Affect Disord* **50**(2–3): 269–76.

Hawton, K. and van Heeringen, K. (2009). Suicide'. *Lancet* **373**(9672): 1372–81.

Hulten, A. and Wasserman, D. (1998). Lack of continuity—a problem in the care of young suicides. *Acta Psychiatr Scand* **97**(5): 326–33.

Kapur, N., Cooper, J., King-Hele, S., et al. (2006). The repetition of suicidal behavior: a multicenter cohort study. *J Clin Psychiatry* **67**(10): 1599–609.

Kessing, L. V. (2004). Severity of depressive episodes according to ICD-10: prediction of risk of relapse and suicide. *Br J Psychiatry* **184**: 153–6.

Marzuk, P. M., Tardiff, K., Leon, A. C., et al. (1995). Use of prescription psychotropic drugs among suicide victims in New York City. *Am J Psychiatry* **152**(10): 1520–2.

The National Confidential Inquiry into Suicide and Homicide by People with Mental Illness (2001). *Safety First: Five-year Report of the National Confidential Inquiry into Suicide and Homicide by People with Mental Illness*. London: Department of Health.

O'Connor, R. C. and Nock, M. K. (2014). The psychology of suicidal behaviour. *Lancet Psychiatry* **1**(1): 73–85.

Phillips, M. R. (2010). Rethinking the role of mental illness in suicide. *Am J Psychiatry* **167**(7): 731–3.

Qin, P., Agerbo, E., and Mortensen, P. B. (2003). Suicide risk in relation to socioeconomic, demographic, psychiatric, and familial factors: a national register-based study of all suicides in Denmark, 1981–1997. *Am J Psychiatry* **160**(4): 765–72.

Qin, P., Hawton, K., Mortensen, P. B., and Webb, R. (2014). Combined effects of physical illness and comorbid psychiatric disorder on risk of suicide in a national population study. *Br J Psychiatry* **204**(6): 430–5.

Siegel, R. L., Jacobs, E. J., Newton, C. C., et al. (2015). Deaths due to cigarette smoking for 12 smoking-related cancers in the United States. *JAMA Intern Med* **175**(9): 1574–6.

Stenager, E. N. and Stenager, E. (2000). Physical illness and suicidal behavior. In *International Handbook of Suicide and Attempted Suicide*, K. Hawton and K. van Heeringen (eds), pp. 405–20. Chichester: John Wiley.

Voracek, M. and Loibl, L. M. (2007). Genetics of suicide: a systematic review of twin studies. *Wien Klin Wochenschr* **119**(15–16): 463–75.

Waern, M., Beskow, J., Runeson, B., and Skoog, I. (1999). Suicidal feelings in the last year of life in elderly people who commit suicide. *Lancet* **354**(9182): 917–18.

Webb, R. T., Kontopantelis, E., Doran, T., Qin, P., Creed, F., and Kapur, N. (2012). Suicide risk in primary care patients with major physical diseases: a case-control study. *Arch Gen Psychiatry* **69**(3): 256–64.

CHAPTER 4

Psychiatric disorders and biological factors

KEY POINTS
• All psychiatric disorders are associated with a high risk of suicide, particularly mood disorders, schizophrenia, and substance misuse.
• Comorbidity is common.
• The vulnerability to suicidal behaviour is partly inherited.
• Serotonin and hypothalamic–pituitary–adrenal axis abnormalities are associated with suicide.
• Biological factors lack specificity for suicide.
• There is an interaction between genetic susceptibility and the environment.

5.1 Psychiatric disorders and suicide

All psychiatric disorders are associated with an elevated risk of suicide. A classic meta-analysis combined the results of 249 studies that had followed up people for at least two years (Harris and Barraclough, 1997); there were over 7,000 deaths by suicide. Table 5.1 summarizes the findings, which are presented as standardized mortality ratios (SMRs). This statistic indicates the mortality rate in the sample of interest when compared to the mortality rate that would be expected in a 'standard population' with a similar age and sex profile. A SMR of 100 indicates equivalent risk while SMRs of greater than 100 indicate increased risk of suicide. Most psychiatric disorders were associated with an increased risk of suicide. Schizophrenia was associated with an eightfold increase in risk, bipolar disorder with a fifteenfold increase in risk, and depression with a twentyfold increase in risk,. Eating disorders also conferred substantially increased risk. All treatment settings (inpatient, community, forensic) were associated with greater risk of suicide, but most studies were carried out in secondary care. These results may therefore not be generalizable to patients receiving treatment for their mental disorder in primary care settings.

In a study in Denmark involving 72,000 individuals followed for up to 20 years, there were nearly 13,000 suicide deaths (Hiroeh et al., 2001). The SMR for those hospitalized with psychiatric disorder was 1356 for women (or over 13 times the expected rate) and 1212 for men (or over 12 times the expected rate). The risks associated with individual disorders in the Danish study were similar to those reported in the meta-analysis, with the exception of the SMRs for alcohol problems and personality disorder, both of which were higher in the Danish study possibly

Table 5.1 Common mental disorders and the risk of suicide (Harris and Barraclough, 1997)

Disorder	SMR (95%CI)
Schizophrenia	845 (798 to 895)
Bipolar disorder	1505 (1225 to 1844)
Major depression	2035 (1827 to 2259)
Dysthymia	1212 (1150 to 1277)
Panic disorder	1000 (457 to 1898)
Alcohol misuse	586 (541 to 633)
Substance use: opiods	1400 (1079 to 1788)
Substance use: hypnotics	2034 (1425 to 2816)
Eating disorders	2314 (1538 to 3344)
Personality disorders	708 (477 to 1010)

SMR: standardized mortality ratio—figures over 100 indicate increased risk of suicide; CI: confidence interval

Adapted from *British Journal of Psychiatry*, 170, Harris EC. and Barraclough B., Suicide as an outcome for mental disorders. A meta-analysis, pp. 205-228. © 1997 The Royal College of Psychiatrists. DOI: https://doi.org/10.1192/bjp.170.3.205

because of the definitions and categories used. (SMR for 'alcoholism': women 1586, men 1064; SMR for personality disorder: women 1568, men 1198.)

In the UK, the National Confidential Inquiry into Suicide and Homicide by Mental Illness has, since 1996, been collecting data on all people who die by suicide within 12 months of psychiatric contact. Figure 5.1 shows the most common psychiatric diagnoses in patients who died by suicide.

5.1.1 Depression

In the Harris and Barraclough review, there were 23 follow-up studies of depressive disorder and nine of dysthymia, which, when analysed, demonstrated that patients with these conditions had a suicide risk of 20 and 12 times, respectively, that of people with no mood disorder. The lifetime risk of suicide associated with major depression is around 3.5 per cent (Blair-West et al., 1997), and psychological autopsy studies have demonstrated that 60–70 per cent of those who die by suicide have symptoms consistent with depressive disorder at the time of death (Cavanagh et al., 2003; Rihmer, 2011).

5.1.1.1 Depression in low- and middle-income countries

Much of the existing research has been carried out in high-income countries. There has been debate about the relative importance of mood disorders in low- and middle-income countries. In some studies it has been reported that 80 per

Patient suicide: primary psychiatric diagnoses (England, 2006-2016)
(source: National Confidential Inquiry into suicide)

Total = 13,187 patients

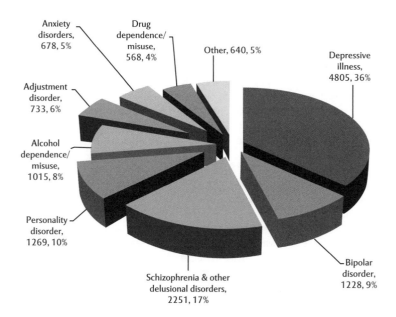

Fig 5.1 Patient suicide: primary psychiatric diagnoses (England, 2006–2016).
Source data: National Confidential Inquiry into Suicide.

cent of those who died by suicide had symptoms consistent with depression be-fore their death (Cheng, 1995). However, depression was reported to be less prominent in a study of people aged 15–24 years from mainland China, where 57 per cent had had depressive symptoms in the two weeks before their death (Li et al., 2008). Of course, the presence of depressive symptoms per se is not necessarily indicative of a formal mental disorder. A recent review reported that psychiatric disorders and depression may be less frequent antecedents of suicide in Asia than in Europe, Australia, and North America, but findings from individual studies were highly variable (Chen et al., 2012). Treatment remains a potentially important preventive strategy in these settings.

5.1.1.2 Under-diagnosis and treatment of depression

A common theme in some studies is that mood disorders were not diagnosed in many who died by suicide, and that even when they were, levels of treatment were inadequate (Rihmer, 2011). One review suggested that only about a third of people who died by suicide had received adequate antidepressant treatment (Isometsa, 2001).

5.1.1.3 Mood disorders in young people

It is sometimes suggested that mood disorders may be of less relevance in suicide in young people. However, a study of 120 young people under 20 years old who died by suicide in New York reported that two thirds had a mood disorder and 50 per cent had a duration of symptoms lasting more than three years. Fewer than 5 per cent had symptoms for less than three months (Shaffer et al., 1996). This study is particularly important as it indicates that there may be a window of opportunity during which the mood disorder could be recognized and treated in young people. However, a larger more recent UK study of young people aged under 20, relying on routine data sources, found that mood disorder was less common, being recorded in about one fifth of cases (Rodway et al., 2016).

5.1.1.4 Depression in self-harm

The association of mood disorders with self-harm and attempted suicide is some-times considered less clear-cut than the association with suicide. Early studies reported that less than 10 per cent of people who attempted suicide had depres-sive conditions, but it became apparent that when standardized instruments were used, more depression was identified than had been the case with clinical reports. A UK study suggested that as many as 90 per cent of self-harm patients may have an axis I psychiatric disorder according to research criteria (Haw et al., 2001). The most common diagnosis in this study was depressive disorder (70 per cent). Almost half of participants had psychiatric comorbidity. However, it is possible that any psychiatric symptoms at the time of an episode are relatively transient and may remit spontaneously in a substantial proportion of people.

5.1.1.5 Depression and suicidal ideation

Suicidal ideation may sometimes be normalized as a phase of life or a readily understood reaction to external stressors. What can be concluded from a number of studies (using definitions as varied as 'life-weariness' or feeling that life is 'not worth living') is that there are high rates of mental disorders, particularly depression, in those endorsing such thoughts. There have also been studies of population burden, which have suggested PARs of depression are similar for sui-cide, attempted suicide, and suicidal ideation (Goldney et al., 2003).

5.1.1.6 Risk factors for suicide in depression

A recent review reported that factors significantly associated with suicide in people who were depressed included a number of conventional risk factors such as male sex, family history of psychiatric disorder, previous history of suicidal be-haviour, severity of depression, hopelessness, and comorbid disorders (such as anxiety and misuse of alcohol and drugs) (Hawton et al., 2013).

5.1.2 Bipolar disorder

A meta-analytic review of 14 reports from seven countries of 3,700 patients found that those with bipolar disorders had a suicide risk 15 times that of those with no disorder (Harris and Barraclough, 1997). Pompili and colleagues suggested that the risk, although highly variable across studies, was approximately 20–30 times that in the general population (Pompili et al., 2013).

In a systematic review, the most important risk factors for suicide in bipolar disorder were a previous attempt and hopelessness (Hawton et al., 2005). For attempted suicide, the risk factors were a family history of suicide, early onset of bipolar disorder, increasing severity of affective episodes, rapid cycling, and comorbidity, particularly with abuse of alcohol and other substances. Another review suggested that the most important clinical risk factors in bipolar disorder included acute symptoms, prior course of illness (e.g. rapid cycling, early onset), personality factors (e.g. aggression, impulsivity), and personal history (childhood adversity, psychosocial stressors, family history) (Pompili et al., 2013). A large UK study found that of nearly 1,500 people with bipolar disorder who had died by suicide, 40 per cent had not been prescribed mood stabilizers (Clements et al., 2013).

5.1.3 Schizophrenia

Bleuler (1911) noted that one of the most serious symptoms of schizophrenia was the 'suicidal drive.' One review found that people with this illness had an eight times higher suicide risk than the general population (Harris and Barraclough, 1997), and another reported around a 5 per cent lifetime risk of dying by suicide (Palmer et al., 2005). Illness-related risk factors (Hor and Taylor, 2010) include:

- Past history of suicide attempts
- Depressive symptoms
- Active delusions and hallucinations
- Having insight into their illness
- Comorbid substance abuse

Social isolation and interpersonal rejection are also often observed prior to suicidal behaviour (Pompili et al., 2007). Adherence to effective treatment is likely to be protective.

5.1.4 The role of alcohol

About 40 per cent of those with alcohol dependence will attempt suicide, and up to 7 per cent will die by suicide (Sher, 2006). Psychological autopsy studies have reported that approximately 15 per cent of women and 30 per cent of men who have died by suicide had potentially diagnosable alcohol dependence.

Disinhibition whilst intoxicated can lead to acts of aggression and impulsivity, increasing the risk of suicidal behavior. Longer-term misuse is associated with depression and chronic suicide risk (Hufford, 2001; Cherpitel et al., 2004; Sher,

2006). Risk is increased for those with comorbid major depression and a previous suicide attempt, and other general risk factors include interpersonal rejection, social isolation, comorbid other substance abuse (particularly cocaine), and a family history of alcohol dependence. Individual risk factors lack specificity and it could be reasonably argued that all those with alcohol dependence should be considered at some risk of suicidal behaviour.

Suicide risk is associated with the availability of alcohol, and there have been suggestions that limiting societal alcohol availability may be an effective suicide prevention measure (Varnik et al., 2007).

5.1.5 Drug misuse

The association of drugs with suicide has been reviewed in an extension of the Harris and Barraclough (1997) meta-analysis of outcome studies (Wilcox et al., 2004). The estimated risks of suicide for alcohol use disorder, opioid use disorder, intravenous drug use, and mixed drug use were 10, 14, 14, and 17 times higher respectively, than those of non-users. It was noted that there were limited data regarding cocaine and cannabis. However, using a different research methodology, it was suggested that most of the modest increased risk in the association of cannabis and serious suicide attempts in a New Zealand sample was related to confounding factors, such as social disadvantage. Cannabis use was comorbid with mental disorders which themselves were independently associated with suicidal behaviour (Beautrais et al., 1999). Similarly, in a French study, cannabis was not associated with life-threatening drug overdoses, whereas use of LSD, buprenorphine, or opiates was (Tournier et al., 2005). However, in a recent twin study from Australia with a large sample, frequent cannabis use (more than 100 times in a lifetime) was associated with a risk of depression and suicidal ideation even after adjustment for confounders (Agrawal et al., 2017).

5.1.6 Personality disorder

The term 'personality disorder' is potentially problematic because it can be stigmatizing and is sometimes used in mental health services as shorthand for hard to engage service users. In research studies, those meeting diagnostic criteria for personality disorders, particularly when comorbid with mood disorders, have an increased risk of suicide (Krysinska et al., 2006). In fact, the criteria for borderline personality disorder include recurrent suicidal behaviour or self-injury. These personality disorders may be associated with a range of early adverse life experiences. Specific interventions for people with so-called personality disorder are discussed in Chapter 9.

5.1.7 Comorbidity

Having more than one psychiatric disorder seems to confer additional risk. In a Finnish psychological autopsy study of 229 people who had died by suicide, the most prevalent axis I diagnosis was a depressive disorder (59 per cent) (Henriksson et al., 1993). However, 43 per cent had alcohol dependence or abuse; 31 per cent had an axis II or personality diagnosis; and 46 per cent had at least one axis III (physical illness) diagnosis. In fact, overall, only 12 per cent of those who died by suicide received one axis I diagnosis without any comorbidity. Comorbidity may more than double the risk of a suicide attempt in people with mood disorder (from 33 times that of people with no mental disorder to 89 times) (Beautrais et al., 1996). Comorbid physical illness also confers additional suicide risk (see Chapter 4). It has been suggested that at least some of the excess suicide risk observed in eating disorders is accounted for by comorbid psychiatric disorder (Yao et al.,2016)

5.2 Genetic influences

There had been clinical observations of an inherited tendency to suicide as long ago as 1790 by Moore (see Chapter 1), but it was not until the 1970s that the hereditary contribution to suicidal behaviour was given a firm scientific basis when a Danish adoption study examined individuals who were separated at birth from their biological relatives (Schulsinger et al., 1979). Using a matched control design, suicide was more common in the biological relatives of the adopted individuals who had died by suicide than in the biological relatives of adopted living controls. Twin studies added to the evidence base. A study of 399 twin pairs demonstrated a 13.2 per cent concordance for suicide in the 129 identical (monozygous) twins, compared with 0.7 per cent concordance for suicide in the 270 non-identical (dizygous) twin pairs (Roy et al., 2000). In another study of 5,995 twins, a logistic regression analysis, which controlled for sociodemographic, personality, psychiatric, trauma, and family history variables, demonstrated that at least 45 per cent of the variance in suicidal thoughts and behaviour was related to genetic factors (Statham et al., 1998). In a recent review, the heritability for suicidal behaviour (the proportion of the variance related to genetic factors) has been estimated as 30–50% (Turecki and Brent, 2016).

A landmark in the recognition of the interrelationship between inherited and environmental factors was research which demonstrated that persons with one or two copies of the short allele of the serotonin T promoter polymorphism experienced more depression and suicidality in response to stressful life events than those who were homozygous for (that is, had two copies of) the long allele (Caspi et al., 2003)—a powerful example of a gene–environment interaction.

Since then, increasingly sophisticated genome analyses have been undertaken (Uher and Perroud, 2010). The results have illustrated the complexity of the challenge, but no specific genes for suicide have yet been identified. However, studies examining impulsive aggression associated with the serotonergic system are promising (Brent, 2009), particularly with an appreciation of gene–environment interactions which may result in a modification of gene expression and activity (Turecki et al., 2012).

It has been suggested that early life adversity may cause long-term effects through changes to gene expression which affect the hypothalamic–pituitary–adrenal (HPA) axis and the stress response (Turecki and Brent, 2016).

5.3 Biochemistry of suicide

5.3.1 Serotonin and other neurotransmitters

An early study found a lowered level of 5-hydroxy indole acetic acid (5-HIAA) in the cerebrospinal fluid (CSF) of suicide attempters who had used violent methods (Asberg et al., 1976). This was important, as CSF 5-HIAA is a breakdown product of serotonin, one of the neurotransmitters associated with mood and behaviour disturbances. This finding has been replicated in different centres, and those people who have attempted suicide, particularly by violent means, and who have a low CSF 5-HIAA, have a greater likelihood of subsequently dying by suicide (Mann and Currier, 2010).

The importance of serotonin transmission has also been demonstrated by post-mortem studies. There is a reduction in serotonin transporter binding in the ventromedial prefrontal cortex and anterior cingulate regions of the brain of those who died by suicide compared with those who died from other causes. The association between suicidal behaviour and the serotonin system is complex. It is unclear to what extent this serotonin dysfunction is specific to people who die by suicide compared to people who are depressed. It may be related to aggression or impulsivity, rather than to any specific psychiatric disorder or suicide per se (Mann and Currier, 2010).

Other neurotransmitters that may be important in suicidal behaviour include gamma-amino butyric acid (GABA). Ketamine, an anaesthetic agent which targets the glutamate pathway, has shown some promise in the acute treatment of people who are suicidal (Reinstatler and Youssef, 2015). The rapid antidepressant and anti-suicidal effects of ketamine are now a major focus of research activity and discussion (Loo, 2018). Polyamines, glial cell factors, and inflammatory processes have also been implicated in the neurobiology of suicide (Turecki and Brent, 2016).

5.3.2 Hypothalamic–pituitary–adrenal axis

There is also evidence of the importance of the hypothalamic–pituitary–adrenal (HPA) axis and the noradrenergic system (Mann and Currier, 2010). A meta-analysis of studies employing the dexamethasone suppression test (DST), which is used to assess functioning of the HPA axis, demonstrated that for non-suppressors compared with suppressors in those with major depression, there was a fourfold higher risk of suicide (Mann et al., 2006). In other words, those in whom the stress response was blunted (that is, the non-suppressors) had a higher risk of suicide. Furthermore, people who were depressed at the time of death had fewer noradrenaline neurons in the locus ceruleus. Other receptor-binding abnormalities have also been reported (Mann and Currier, 2010). A more recent meta-analysis suggested that there was a positive correlation between serum cortisol (a stress hormone) and suicidal behaviour in people aged under 40 years and a negative correlation in older people (O'Connor et al., 2016). This could be accounted for by the concept of allostatic load—repeated activation of the HPA axis through stress eventually leads to dysregulation in later years.

5.4 Neuropsychological deficits

Neuropsychological deficits in those with suicidal behaviour have been reported, with general executive function, decision making, visual memory, and verbal fluency deficits linked to dorsolateral prefrontal and orbitofrontal regions of the brain (LeGris and van Reekum, 2006). People with suicidal behaviour may focus on suicidal thoughts (deficits in attentional shifting), have difficulty communicating a need for help (deficits in verbal fluency), and may be prone to impulsive and risky behaviour (poor decision making) (Bolton et al., 2015).

5.5 Conclusion

Psychiatric disorders, biological factors, and genetic factors increase the risk of suicidal behaviour, and may increase the susceptibility of some individuals to react more severely to stress, but do not inevitably lead to suicide. They should not detract from the central role of an individual's experience in his or her psychosocial environment. It is clear that mental disorders and biological factors are important in their own right and should be integrated into suicide prevention programmes. Figure 5.2 is an infographic summarizing the information in this chapter.

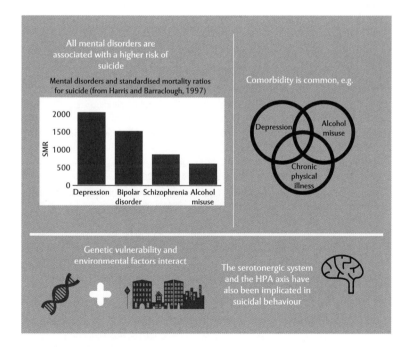

Fig 5.2 **Mental disorders and suicide.**
Courtesy of Dr Sarah Steeg.

REFERENCES

Agrawal, A., Nelson, E. C., Bucholz, K. K., et al. (2017). Major depressive disorder, suicidal thoughts and behaviours, and cannabis involvement in discordant twins: a retrospective cohort study. *Lancet Psychiatry* **4**(9): 706–14.

Asberg, M., Traskman, L., and Thoren, P. (1976). 5-HIAA in the cerebrospinal fluid. A biochemical suicide predictor? *Arch Gen Psychiatry* **33**(10): 1193–7.

Beautrais, A. L., Joyce, P. R., and Mulder, R. T. (1999). Cannabis abuse and serious suicide attempts. *Addiction* **94**(8): 1155–64.

Beautrais, A. L., Joyce, P. R., Mulder, R. T., Fergusson, D. M., Deavoll, B. J., and Nightingale, S. K. (1996). Prevalence and comorbidity of mental disorders in persons making serious suicide attempts: a case-control study. *Am J Psychiatry* **153**(8): 1009–14.

Blair-West, G. W., Mellsop, G. W., and Eyeson-Annan, M. L. (1997). Down-rating lifetime suicide risk in major depression. *Acta Psychiatr Scand* **95**(3): 259–63.

Bleuler, E. (1911) (1950). *Dementia Praecox or the Group of Schizophrenias*, trans. by J. Zinkin, p. 488. New York: International Universities Press.

Bolton, J. M., Gunnell, D., and Turecki, G. (2015). Suicide risk assessment and intervention in people with mental illness. *BMJ* **351**: h4978.

Brent, D. (2009). In search of endophenotypes for suicidal behavior. *Am J Psychiatry* **166**(10): 1087–9.

Caspi, A., K. Sugden, T. E. Moffitt, A. Taylor, I. W. Craig, H. Harrington, J. McClay, J. Mill, J. Martin, A. Braithwaite and R. Poulton (2003). 'Influence of life stress on depression: moderation by a polymorphism in the 5-HTT gene'. *Science* **301**(5631): 386–389.

Cavanagh, J. T., Carson, A. J., Sharpe, M., and Lawrie, S. M. (2003). Psychological autopsy studies of suicide: a systematic review. *Psychol Med* **33**(3): 395–405.

Chen, Y. Y., Wu, K. C., Yousuf, S., and Yip, P. S. (2012). Suicide in Asia: opportunities and challenges. *Epidemiol Rev* **34**: 129–44.

Cheng, A. T. (1995). Mental illness and suicide. A case-control study in east Taiwan. *Arch Gen Psychiatry* **52**(7): 594–603.

Cherpitel, C. J., Borges, G. L., and Wilcox, H. C. (2004). Acute alcohol use and suicidal behavior: a review of the literature. *Alcohol Clin Exp Res* **28**(5 Suppl): 18S–28S.

Clements, C., Morriss, R., Jones, S., Peters, S., Roberts, C., and Kapur, N. (2013). Suicide in bipolar disorder in a national English sample, 1996–2009: frequency, trends and characteristics. *Psychol Med* **43**(12): 2593–602.

Goldney, R. D., Dal Grande, E., Fisher, L. J., and Wilson, D. (2003). Population attributable risk of major depression for suicidal ideation in a random and representative community sample. *J Affect Disord* **74**(3): 267–72.

Harris, E. C. and Barraclough, B. (1997). Suicide as an outcome for mental disorders. A meta-analysis. *Br J Psychiatry* **170**: 205–28.

Haw, C., Hawton, K., Houston, K., and Townsend, E. (2001). Psychiatric and personality disorders in deliberate self-harm patients. *Br J Psychiatry* **178**(1): 48–54.

Hawton, K., Casanas, I. C. C., Haw, C., and Saunders, K. (2013). Risk factors for suicide in individuals with depression: a systematic review. *J Affect Disord* **147**(1–3): 17–28.

CHAPTER 5

Hawton, K., Sutton, L., Haw, C., Sinclair, J., and Harriss, L. (2005). Suicide and attempted suicide in bipolar disorder: a systematic review of risk factors. *J Clin Psychiatry* **66**(6): 693–704.

Henriksson, M. M., Aro, H. M., Marttunen, M. J., et al. (1993). Mental disorders and comorbidity in suicide. *Am J Psychiatry* **150**(6): 935–40.

Hiroeh, U., Appleby, L., Mortensen, P. B., and Dunn, G. (2001). Death by homicide, suicide, and other unnatural causes in people with mental illness: a population-based study. *Lancet* **358**(9299): 2110–12.

Hor, K. and Taylor, M. (2010). Suicide and schizophrenia: a systematic review of rates and risk factors. *J Psychopharmacol* **24**(4 Suppl): 81–90.

Hufford, M. R. (2001). Alcohol and suicidal behavior. *Clin Psychol Rev* **21**(5): 797–811.

Isometsa, E. T. (2001). Psychological autopsy studies—a review. *Eur Psychiatry* **16**(7): 379–85.

Krysinska, K., Heller, T. S., and De Leo, D. (2006). Suicide and deliberate self-harm in personality disorders. *Curr Opin Psychiatry* **19**(1): 95–101.

LeGris, J. and van Reekum, R. (2006). The neuropsychological correlates of borderline personality disorder and suicidal behaviour. *Can J Psychiatry* **51**(3): 131–42.

Li, X. Y., Phillips, M. R., Zhang, Y. P., Xu, D., and Yang, G. H. (2008). Risk factors for suicide in China's youth: a case-control study. *Psychol Med* **38**(3): 397–406.

Loo, C. (2018). Can we confidently use ketamine as a clinical treatment for depression? *Lancet Psychiatry* **5**(1): 11–12.

Mann, J. J., Currier, D., Stanley, B., Oquendo, M. A., Amsel, L. V., and Ellis, S. P. (2006). Can biological tests assist prediction of suicide in mood disorders? *Int J Neuropsychopharmacol* **9**(4): 465–74.

Mann, J. J. and Currier, D. M. (2010). Stress, genetics and epigenetic effects on the neurobiology of suicidal behavior and depression. *Eur Psychiatry* **25**(5): 268–71.

O'Connor, D. B., Ferguson, E., Green, J. A., O'Carroll, R. E., and O'Connor, R. C. (2016). Cortisol levels and suicidal behavior: a meta-analysis. *Psychoneuroendocrinology* **63**: 370–9.

Palmer, B. A., Pankratz, V. S., and Bostwick, J. M. (2005). The lifetime risk of suicide in schizophrenia: a reexamination. *Arch Gen Psychiatry* **62**(3): 247–53.

Pompili, M., Amador, X. F., Girardi, P., et al. (2007). Suicide risk in schizophrenia: learning from the past to change the future. *Ann Gen Psychiatry* **6**: 10.

Pompili, M., Gonda, X., Serafini, G., et al. (2013). Epidemiology of suicide in bipolar disorders: a systematic review of the literature. *Bipolar Disord* **15**(5): 457–90.

Reinstatler, L. and Youssef, N. A. (2015). Ketamine as a potential treatment for suicidal ideation: a systematic review of the literature. *Drugs R D* **15**(1): 37–43.

Rihmer, Z. (2011). Depression and suicidal behaviour. In *The International Handbook of Suicide Prevention: Research, Policy and Practice*, R. C. O'Connor, S. Platt, and J. Gordon (eds), pp. 59–74. Chichester: Wiley-Blackwell.

Rodway, C., Tham, S. G., Ibrahim, S., et al. (2016). Suicide in children and young people in England: a consecutive case series. *Lancet Psychiatry* **3**(8): 751–9.

Roy, A., Nielsen, D., Rylander, G., and Sarchiapone, M. (2000). The genetics of suicidal behaviour. In *The International Handbook of Suicide and Attempted Suicide*, K. Hawton and K. van Heeringen (eds), pp. 209–22. Chichester: John Wiley.

Schulsinger, F., Kety, S. S., Rosenthal, D., and Wender, P. H. (1979). A family study of suicide. In *Origin, Prevention and Treatment of Affective Disorders*, M. Schou and E. Stromgren (eds), pp. 277–87 . London: Academic Pres.

Shaffer, D., Gould, M. S., Fisher, P., et al. (1996). Psychiatric diagnosis in child and adolescent suicide. *Arch Gen Psychiatry* **53**(4): 339–48.

Sher, L. (2006). Risk and protective factors for suicide in patients with alcoholism. *Sci World J* **6**: 1405–11.

Statham, D. J., Heath, A. C., Madden, P. A., et al. (1998). Suicidal behaviour: an epidemiological and genetic study. *Psychol Med* **28**(4): 839–55.

Tournier, M., Molimard, M., Abouelfath, A., et al. (2005). Prognostic impact of psychoactive substances use during hospitalization for intentional drug overdose. *Acta Psychiatr Scand* **112**(2): 134–40.

Turecki, G. and Brent, D. A. (2016). Suicide and suicidal behaviour. *Lancet* **387**(10024): 1227–39.

Turecki, G., Ernst, C., Jollant, F., Labonte, B., and Mechawar, N. (2012). The neurodevelopmental origins of suicidal behavior. *Trends Neurosci* **35**(1): 14–23.

Uher, R. and Perroud, N. (2010). Probing the genome to understand suicide. *Am J Psychiatry* **167**(12): 1425–7.

Varnik, A., Kolves, K., Vali, M., Tooding, L. M., and Wasserman, D. (2007). Do alcohol restrictions reduce suicide mortality? *Addiction* **102**(2): 251–6.

Wilcox, H. C., Conner, K. R., and Caine, E. D. (2004). Association of alcohol and drug use disorders and completed suicide: an empirical review of cohort studies. *Drug Alcohol Depend* **76 Suppl**: S11–19.

Yao, S., Kuja-Halkola, R., Thornton, L. M., Runfola, C. D., D'Onofrio, B. M., Almqvist, C., Lichtenstein, P., Sjölander, A., Larsson, H., Bulik, C. M. (2016). Familial Liability for Eating Disorders and Suicide Attempts: Evidence From a Population Registry in Sweden. *JAMA Psychiatry*. doi:10.1001/jamapsychiatry.2015.2737. Published online January 13, 2016

CHAPTER 5

Psychosocial and societal influences on suicidal behaviour

KEY POINTS

- Broad societal influences on suicidal behaviour—such as employment and other socioeconomic factors, social integration, and religion—are important.
- The prominence they have been given has fluctuated over time.
- Diverse developmental factors have also been associated with suicide.
- Adverse life events, particularly interpersonal conflict, often precede suicidal behaviour.
- Situational factors, such as the media and access to means of suicide, also contribute.
- Interpersonal-psychological theories can shed further light on our understanding of suicidal behaviour.

6.1 Introduction

The presumed importance of broad psychosocial influences, as opposed to individual factors, in contributing to suicidal behaviours has fluctuated over time. Early nineteenth-century authors suggested that suicide was caused by an interplay of factors. However, following this there was an increasing focus on sociological causes, which culminated in Durkheim's seminal work. Views of suicide both as a complex behaviour with a varied aetiology and as a socially driven phenomenon retain a contemporary relevance.

6.2 Broad psychosocial and societal influences

Mid-nineteenth-century authors emphasized the importance of societal organization and specific social problems. The influence of civil status, occupation, and literacy were also well recognized. 'Altruistic' and 'egotistical' suicide had been described by Savage in 1892, prior to Durkheim's more widely known sociological theory, including his description of anomic, egoistic, altruistic, and fatalistic suicide (Goldney et al., 2008) (see Box 6.1). Suicidal behaviour in this model was not viewed as an individual phenomenon but as a function of the relationship between the individual and the wider community (that is, a function of social integration).

During the twentieth century, psychosocial influences were explored extensively. Factors such as socioeconomic and civil status, unemployment, social

> **Box 6.1** Durkheim and suicidal behaviour
>
> **Altruistic suicide**—ending one's life for the sake of the wider group, the greater good.
> **Fatalistic suicide**—occurs as a consequence of the overly strict rules of a society impairing individual freedom.
> **Egoistic suicide**—may occur in situations where the individual no longer feels a sense of community and consequently does not feel bound by societal norms.
> **Anomic suicide**—reflects a situation in which perhaps at a time of societal upheaval, the ability of the community to create and maintain social norms is inadequate and its ability to exercise social control insufficient.

organization, social integration, and religion were noted to be associated with suicidal behaviour. Psychosocial causes of suicide may have been most apparent in those countries or regions which had high or rapidly changing suicide rates. For example, it was considered that the communist oppression of personal freedom in Eastern European countries contributed to their high rates of suicide. During the first years of increasing freedom under 'Perestroika', there was a reduction of suicide in the former USSR (Varnik et al., 1998). However, in the 1990s, suicide rates in those countries increased again and the WHO observed that from the sociopolitical perspective, political reforms which led to western-orientated changes may have caused economic and political problems and distress for many (WHO, 1999). A further example is the phenomenon of relatively high female suicide rates in rural China in the recent past, which was considered to be related to unique psychosocial pressures on females in modern Chinese society. However, that is changing, with greater parity between genders and higher rates of suicide in males (Li et al., 2012; Wang et al., 2014). It is also important to note that the ready availability of lethal organophosphate pesticides has probably contributed to the high female suicide rate in China, just as it has in other countries such as Sri Lanka and Western Samoa. However, even in these settings lower socioeconomic position is associated with an increased risk of suicidal behaviour (Knipe et al., 2015).

Perhaps less commonly discussed are the extremely low rates of suicide in some countries. Such rates may be a reflection of inconsistent recording, poor quality statistics, or a result of stigma. In some countries, there are still sanctions against the reporting of suicide or suicide may even be illegal (WHO, 2014). Traditionally, the example of Roman Catholic Ireland has been used to illustrate the under-reporting of suicide. The historically low rates for Ireland seemed unlikely, and careful enquiry about religious influence and coronial practices indicated that the true rate was appreciably greater than had hitherto been reported (Goldney, 2010). More recently, very low rates of suicide have been reported from some Islamic countries (Shah and Chandia, 2010). For religions which prohibit suicide, there may be stigma which results in reduced reporting. However, on an individual level, religious observance may be protective against suicidal behaviour (Lawrence et al., 2016).

6.3 Unemployment and economic factors

Economic factors may be a key determinant of population mental health and therefore suicide rates. Stuckler and colleagues, in a study of 26 European countries, found that for every 1 per cent increase in unemployment during a recession there was a 0.79 per cent increase in suicide (Stuckler et al., 2009).

The global economic downturn of 2008 may have had important effects on the rate of suicide. A study of 54 countries worldwide reported nearly 5,000 excess deaths in 2009 compared to the numbers that would be expected based on trends prior to the recession (Chang et al., 2013). In men, rates were 4 per cent higher than expected in Europe and 6 per cent higher in the USA (see Figure 6.1).

Unemployment is not the only economic indicator which may have an impact. Whilst it is clearly important, especially in men in mid life, factors such as personal

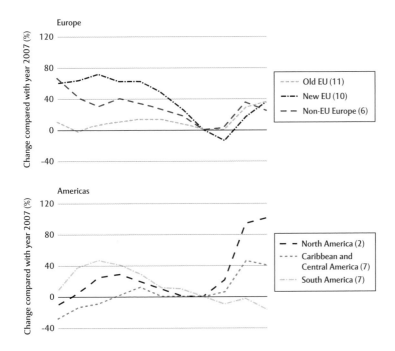

Fig 6.1 Suicide and recession.

Reproduced from *BMJ*, 347, Chang SS., Stuckler D., Yip P., and Gunnell D., Impact of 2008 global economic crisis on suicide: time trend study in 54 countries. Copyright © 2013, British Medical Journal Publishing Group. doi: https://doi.org/10.1136/bmj.f5239.

debt and house repossession may have more of a role in younger individuals (Coope et al., 2014). Intriguingly, some research suggests that welfare spending and active labour-market programmes may protect people against suicide: in one study, every US$10 per person spent in this way reduced the effect of unemployment on suicides by 0•038 per cent (Stuckler et al., 2009).

6.4 Developmental factors

Various studies have demonstrated the importance of developmental factors (see Box 6.2) in contributing to the propensity to suicidal behaviour in subsequent years (Dube et al., 2001; Fergusson et al., 2003). Abuse in childhood may be particularly important. A recent review suggested that sexual abuse was an important antecedent to suicidal behaviour but that physical abuse and domestic violence were also associated with self-harm (Ford and Gomez, 2015). However, the risk factors are broad, lack specificity, and are related to the development of mental disorders in general (van Heeringen et al., 2000). It seems likely that adverse childhood experiences can lead to later suicidal behaviour but this effect may be partly mediated through an association with clinical factors such as psychiatric disorder.

Other interesting findings include lower weight gain in infancy being associated with suicide in adult life (Barker et al., 1995); suicide risk being increased in those with poor childhood and adolescent physical development, nocturnal enuresis to the age of 4, and in those adolescents who had excessive tics, aggression, or conduct problems and greater emotional instability (Neeleman et al., 1998); lower IQ at age 13 being associated with increased risk for males, but not females (Andersson et al., 2008); and increased height being associated with a decreased incidence of suicide (Magnusson et al., 2005). More recent work has not found an association with height but has reported a consistent inverse association with body mass index (BMI): people with a higher BMI are at reduced risk of suicide (Bjerkeset et al., 2008). The possible mechanisms behind this association include carbohydrate intake, fatty acid and cholesterol metabolism, impaired insulin sensitivity, and cerebral serotonin and tryptophan levels (Klinitzke et al., 2013).

Clearly, many of these issues straddle the psychosocial and biological contributions to suicide, and the findings do not have an easy causal explanation. There are no simple conclusions in considering the impact of developmental issues on the

---

Box 6.2 Developmental factors

- Neo-natal influences
- Parental violence, separation
- Child abuse, particularly sexual but also physical and emotional
- Poor peer relationships
- Bullying
- Educational failure.

---

risk of later suicide. There has been significant recent focus on the link between autism spectrum conditions and suicide risk (Cassidy et al., 2017).

6.5 Life events and situational factors

At the individual level, adverse life events very often precede suicidal behaviour. In addition, the context in which the behaviour occurs is important. Ready access to the means of suicide increases risk, particularly for those who might be prone to impulsive behaviour. Some people are likely to be influenced by media reports.

6.5.1 Adverse life events

It has long been accepted that adverse life events are associated with suicide. Indeed, one review reported a general consensus from worldwide psychological autopsy studies that interpersonal conflict was the most important 'proximal' event (that is, occurring shortly before death) (Foster, 2011). Such conflict was related to separation or less severe issues with partners, peers, or parents. Other life events relate to financial distress, forensic issues, employment, and accommodation. Not unexpectedly, there is evidence of a dose–response effect (those with more life events are at greater risk), but it is of note that adverse life events may have less of a role in the aetiology of suicide in those with severe mental disorders (Cooper et al., 2002).

6.5.2 Access to means of suicide

The likelihood of suicide is influenced by factors such as the provision of natural gas as opposed to coal gas, the availability of firearms, being in a rural environment with pesticides, being in proximity to railways, bridges, and other high frequency locations, and the availability of certain medications (Yip et al., 2012). Addressing the issue of access to means has emerged as one of the most important suicide prevention measures. This will be discussed in detail in Chapter 12.

6.5.3 Imitative suicide

The potential influence of publicity about suicide has been noted for over two hundred years. Concern about imitative suicide led to the banning of Goethe's novel *The Sorrows of Young Werther* in some European countries in the eighteenth century (Phillips, 1974), and, in 1841, William Farr stated that 'no fact is better established in science than that suicide (and murder may perhaps be added) is often committed from imitation' (quoted by Motto, 1967). Despite the strength of that assertion, it took over a hundred years before there was convincing research evidence to confirm it. The phenomenon is presumed to be based on social learning theory and identification with the person who has died by suicide. The effect may be stronger when it is a celebrity who has died by suicide, and the risk may be higher in those who are of a similar age and gender to the celebrity, and use a similar method (Niederkrotenthaler et al., 2012).

Gould categorized the factors which influence the association between media coverage and suicidal behaviour as related to the characteristics of the stories (agent), individuals' attributes (host), and the social context of the stories (environment) (Gould, 2001). Examples of how this relates to prevention will be presented in Chapter 11.

6.6 Psychological theories

6.6.1 Traditional psychoanalytic theories

Traditional Freudian psychoanalytic theory about suicidal behaviour suggests that it is a reaction to the loss of an ambivalently regarded loved object, with the mixed aggressive feelings being turned inward, rather than being externalized, so much so that suicide has been referred to as 'murder in the 180th degree'. Other early theories included that of Stekel, who suggested that nobody killed themselves unless they had wished for the death of someone else; Menninger focused on the wish to die, the wish to kill, and the wish to be killed; and object relations theory posits ego-splitting, with the wish to kill the introjected object (Williams and Pollock, 2000).

6.6.2 Other psychological theories

A 'pre-suicidal syndrome' has been described, in which a constriction of emotion and higher cognitive functioning leads to a narrowing of the range of options (Sonneck, 1986). Suicidal behaviour has also been regarded as a 'cry for help', and in that sense some have suggested it might be interpreted as adaptive from an ethological perspective (Farberow and Shneidman, 1961). These descriptions are consistent with more recent cognitive theories, which have focused on hopelessness and a sense of 'entrapment' (Williams et al., 2005). Entrapment is the inability to avoid a noxious environment after a loss or humiliation. Recent research has indicated that such feelings can be reactivated by inducing a depressed mood. Suicidal ideation then emerges. This cognitive understanding has the potential for the development of specific interventions. For a fuller discussion of more contemporary psychological models, see Chapter 4.

6.6.3 Insights from psychotherapy

Insights from the psychotherapeutic treatment of people with suicidal thoughts or behaviours have provided further understanding. Suicidal behaviour is an intensely personal phenomenon, and the emotional pain associated with it has been referred to as 'psychache' (Shneidman, 1993) or, over one hundred years previously, as 'moral suffering' (Morselli, 1881). Each suicidal person has his or her own view of the world, which frequently becomes constricted so that alternatives to suicide, or at the very least to seeking temporary oblivion, appear remote. The final act is often precipitated by loss of an interpersonal relationship, and there may sometimes be thoughts of retribution or retaliation (Maddison and Mackey, 1966). There may be other thoughts of reunion with significant others who have died, particularly if their death was by suicide. Some writers have talked about the loss of empathy when people are in suicidal despair. The pain and desire to escape means that the person is unable to imagine the distress and feelings of loss in others if they take their own lives (Williams, 2014).

A detailed analysis of those who died by suicide and who had had at least six sessions of psychotherapy suggested that the precipitating event almost invariably occurred in the setting of one or more intense affective states in addition to depression, and they included feelings of desperation, abandonment, and humiliation (Hendin et al., 2007). There were also at least one of three behavioural patterns prior to the suicide: talking about suicide, a reduction in social and/or occupational functioning. and increasing substance abuse.

6.7 Conclusion

Broad societal influences, life events (both early and late), situational factors such as access to means, and media portrayal all influence suicidal behaviour. Psychological theories can help to improve our understanding. Broader influences and a theoretical perspective provide a helpful context and can inform population-level preventive strategies. Figure 6.2 is an infographic summarizing the information in this chapter.

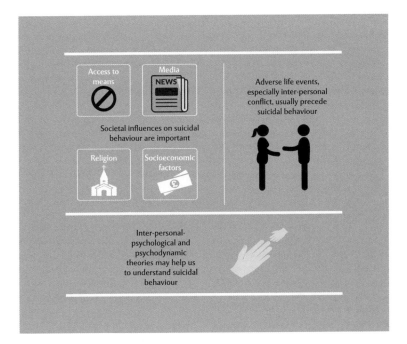

Fig 6.2 Psychosocial and societal influences on suicidal behaviour.
Courtesy of Dr Sarah Steeg.

REFERENCES

Andersson, L., Allebeck, P., Gustafsson, J. E., and Gunnell, D. (2008). Association of IQ scores and school achievement with suicide in a 40-year follow-up of a Swedish cohort. *Acta Psychiatr Scand* **118**(2): 99–105.

Barker, D. J., Osmond, C., Rodin, I., Fall, C. H., and Winter, P. D. (1995). Low weight gain in infancy and suicide in adult life. *BMJ* **311**(7014): 1203.

Bjerkeset, O., Romundstad, P., Evans, J., and Gunnell, D. (2008). Association of adult body mass index and height with anxiety, depression, and suicide in the general population: the HUNT study. *Am J Epidemiol* **167**(2): 193–202.

Cassidy, S., Bradley, P., Robinson, J., Allison, C., McHugh, M., and Baron-Cohen, S. (2014). Suicidal ideation and suicide plans or attempts in adults with Asperger's syndrome attending a specialist diagnostic clinic: a clinical cohort study. *Lancet Psychiatry* **1**: 142–7.

Chang, S. S., Stuckler, D., Yip, P., and Gunnell, D. (2013). Impact of 2008 global economic crisis on suicide: time trend study in 54 countries. *BMJ* **347**: 5239.

Coope, C., Gunnell, D., Hollingworth, W., et al. (2014). Suicide and the 2008 economic recession: who is most at risk? Trends in suicide rates in England and Wales 2001–2011. *Soc Sci Med* **117**: 76–85.

Cooper, J., Appleby, L., and Amos, T. (2002). Life events preceding suicide by young people. *Soc Psychiatry Psychiatr Epidemiol* **37**(6): 271–5.

Dube, S. R., Anda, R. F., Felitti, V. J., Chapman, D. P., Williamson, D. F., and Giles, W. H. (2001). Childhood abuse, household dysfunction, and the risk of attempted suicide throughout the life span: findings from the Adverse Childhood Experiences Study. *JAMA* **286**(24): 3089–96.

Farberow, N. L. and Shneidman, E. S. (1961). *The Cry for Help*. New York: McGraw-Hill.

Fergusson, D. M., Beautrais, A. L., and Horwood, L. J. (2003). Vulnerability and resiliency to suicidal behaviours in young people. *Psychol Med* **33**(1): 61–73.

Ford, J. D. and Gomez, J. M. (2015). The relationship of psychological trauma and dissociative and posttraumatic stress disorders to nonsuicidal self-injury and suicidality: a review. *J Trauma Dissociation* **16**(3): 232–71.

Foster, T. (2011). Adverse life events proximal to adult suicide: a synthesis of findings from psychological autopsy studies. *Arch Suicide Res* **15**(1): 1–15.

Goldney, R. D. (2010). A note on the reliability and validity of suicide statistics. *Psychiatr Psychol Law* **17**(1): 52–6.

Goldney, R. D., Schioldann, J. A., and Dunn, K. I. (2008). Suicide research before Durkheim. *Health History* **10**(2): 73–93.

Gould, M. S. (2001). Suicide and the media. *Ann N Y Acad Sci* **932**: 200–21.

Hendin, H., Maltsberger, J. T., and Szanto, K. (2007). The role of intense affective states in signaling a suicide crisis. *J Nerv Ment Dis* **195**(5): 363–8.

Klinitzke, G., Steinig, J., Bluher, M., Kersting, A., and Wagner, B. (2013). Obesity and suicide risk in adults—a systematic review. *J Affect Disord* **145**(3): 277–84.

Knipe, D. W., Carroll, R., Thomas, K. H., Pease, A., Gunnell, D., and Metcalfe, C. (2015). Association of socio-economic position and suicide/attempted suicide in low and middle income countries in South and South-East Asia—a systematic review. *BMC Public Health* **15**: 1055.

Lawrence, R. E., Oquendo, M. A., and Stanley, B. (2016). Religion and suicide risk: a systematic review. *Arch Suicide Res* **20**(1): 1–21.

Li, Y., Li, Y., and Cao, J. (2012). Factors associated with suicidal behaviors in mainland China: a meta-analysis. *BMC Public Health* **12**: 524.

Maddison, D. and Mackey, K. H. (1966). Suicide: the clinical problem. *Br J Psychiatry* **112**(488): 693–703.

Magnusson, P. K., Gunnell, D., Tynelius, P., Davey Smith, G., and Rasmussen, F. (2005). Strong inverse association between height and suicide in a large cohort of Swedish men: evidence of early life origins of suicidal behavior? *Am J Psychiatry* **162**(7): 1373–5.

Morselli, E. (1881). *Suicide. An Essay on Comparative Moral Statistics.* Revised and abridged by the author for the English version. London: C. Kegan Paul.

Motto, J. A. (1967). Suicide and suggestibility—the role of the press. *Am J Psychiatry* **124**(2): 252–6.

Neeleman, J., Wessely, S., and Wadsworth, M. (1998). Predictors of suicide, accidental death, and premature natural death in a general-population birth cohort. *Lancet* **351**(9096): 93–7.

Niederkrotenthaler, T., Fu, K. W., Yip, P. S., et al. (2012). Changes in suicide rates following media reports on celebrity suicide: a meta-analysis. *J Epidemiol Community Health* **66**(11): 1037–42.

Phillips, D. P. (1974). The influence of suggestion on suicide: substantive and theoretical implications of the Werther effect. *Am Sociol Rev* **39**(3): 340–54.

Shah, A. and Chandia, M. (2010). The relationship between suicide and Islam: a cross-national study. *J Inj Violence Res* **2**(2): 93–7.

Shneidman, E. S. (1993). Suicide as psychache. *J Nerv Ment Dis* **181**(3): 145–7.

Sonneck, G. (1986). On the phenomenology and nosology of the presuicidal syndrome. *Crisis* **7**(2): 111–17.

Stuckler, D., Basu, S., Suhrcke, M., Coutts, A., and McKee, M. (2009). The public health effect of economic crises and alternative policy responses in Europe: an empirical analysis. *Lancet* **374**(9686): 315–23.

van Heeringen, K., Hawton, K., and Williams, J. M. G. (2000). Pathways to suicide: an integrative approach. In *The International Handbook of Suicide and Attempted Suicide*, K. van Heeringen and K. Hawton (eds), pp. 223–36. Chichester: John Wiley.

Varnik, A., Wasserman, D., Dankowicz, M., and Eklund, G. (1998). Marked decrease in suicide among men and women in the former USSR during perestroika. *Acta Psychiatr Scand Suppl* **394**: 13–19.

Wang, C. W., Chan, C. L., and Yip, P. S. (2014). Suicide rates in China from 2002 to 2011: an update. *Soc Psychiatry Psychiatr Epidemiol* **49**(6): 929–41.

Williams, J. M. G. (2014). *Cry of Pain: Understanding Suicide and the Suicidal Mind.* London: Piatkus.

Williams, J. M. G., Crane, C., Barnhofer, T., and Duggan, D. (2005). Psychology and suicidal behaviour: elaborating the entrapment model. In *Prevention and Treatment of Suicidal Behaviour*, K. Hawton (ed.), pp. 71–90. Oxford: Oxford University Press.

Williams, J. M. G. and Pollock, L. R. (2000). Psychology of suicidal behaviour. In *The International Handbook of Suicide and Attempted Suicide*, K. van Heeringen and K. Hawton (eds), pp. 79–93 . Chichester: John Wiley.

World Health Organization (2014). *Preventing Suicide: A Global Imperative 2014.* From http://www.who.int/mental_health/suicide-prevention/world_report_2014/en/

World Health Organization (1999). *Figures and Facts About Suicide.* From http://www.who.int/iris/handle/10665/66097

Yip, P. S., Caine, E., Yousuf, S., Chang, S. S., Wu K. C., and Chen, Y. Y. (2012). Means restriction for suicide prevention. *Lancet* **379**(9834): 2393–9.

CHAPTER 6

CHAPTER 7

Initial assessment and management

KEY POINTS

- The challenges of studying suicidal behaviour and the limitations of research mean that some aspects of assessment have to be pragmatic rather than strictly evidence-based.
- Clinicians should establish rapport early on in assessment.
- Assess suicidal intent.
- Enquire about access to means of suicide.
- Assess mental state.
- A good assessment may be therapeutic in itself.
- If there are interpersonal or other issues and no psychiatric disorder, offer follow-up and problem-solving approaches as appropriate.
- If a psychiatric disorder is present, initiate the relevant treatment for that disorder.
- Consider offering formal psychological interventions to all those who present.

7.1 Limitations of the evidence base

The emphasis on rigorous evidence-based practice in the latter part of the twentieth century led to serious questions being posed about suicide prevention strategies. Researchers pointed out that no specific interventions had proven efficacy for reducing suicide in randomized controlled trials (RCTs) (Gunnell and Frankel, 1994). Reviews of the treatment literature (Hawton et al., 1998) suggested an insufficient evidence base on which to make firm recommendations. However, recent systematic reviews have been more promising, particularly with respect to psychological interventions reducing repeat episodes of self-harm (Hawton et al., 2016; Hetrick et al., 2016).

7.1.1 The low base rate of suicide

Every suicide death is an individual tragedy but the comparatively low base rate of suicide, together with the large number of false positives that result from use of conventional suicide risk factors, mean that we do not have reliable predictors of suicide on an individual level. We discuss this further in the next chapter. The low incidence also imposes limitations on the research methodologies that can be used to demonstrate the effectiveness of specific treatments. For example, to demonstrate a 15 per cent reduction in suicide in those discharged from psychiatric hospitals, assuming there is a 0.9 per cent incidence of suicide in the subsequent year, would require over 140,000 patients in the research sample (Gunnell and Frankel, 1994). The numbers required to demonstrate the effectiveness of the prevention of repetition of attempted suicide are smaller than for suicide, but still considerable. The other challenge is that people recruited to trials may not be representative of the wider clinical population.

7.1.2 The need for alternative research methodologies and a practical approach

The evidence base from systematic reviews of RCTs is somewhat limited and so those with responsibility for suicide prevention could be forgiven for being pessimistic. However, alternative research designs can provide useful information and clinical experience ('practice-based evidence') is often invaluable at an individual patient level.

Cohort designs, before and after studies, even ecological designs can be helpful. Of course, such observational studies cannot demonstrate causation, but newer approaches to address confounding (such as propensity scores and instrumental variable analysis) can be used to help estimate treatment effects from observational data (Carroll et al., 2016; Steeg et al., 2018).

When a more pragmatic approach is taken and searches are widened to include other research designs as well as RCTs, there is a considerable body of evidence which can give professionals some confidence in the practical approaches they can take to reduce suicidal behaviour (Goldney, 2005).

In the end though, not every aspect of the assessment of people presenting in distress with suicidal behaviour will be strongly evidence-based. Some of the framework described here is based on clinical consensus and may need to be adapted according to the individual, the treatment setting, and the wider cultural or national context. Not all health or social care professionals will be providing on-going management to those with suicidal thoughts or behaviours. However, we would argue that all such professionals should have some capacity for conducting the initial assessment and, if indicated, for making recommendations for further management. There are a number of articles which outline assessment by non-specialists (e.g. Morriss et al., 2013). In mental health settings, the assessment of a person who is suicidal has been described as one of the most complex assessments in psychiatry (Isacsson and Rich, 2001). In the UK, work is ongoing to develop a key set of competencies for professionals who assess people who present with suicidal thoughts or behaviour (National Collaborating Centre for Mental Health, 2018).

Fundamental to assessing and managing a suicidal person is to first deal with any serious physical health needs (e.g. treating the after-effects of an overdose, managing lacerations). Thereafter, a psychosocial assessment needs to be carried out in all patients to establish rapport, to assess suicidal intent, and to determine if there is a psychiatric disorder which requires on-going management. But even if there is no clearly defined mental disorder, follow-up support should be offered. Some national guidelines helpfully refer to the aim of the assessment as being to establish the needs of the service user (National Collaborating Centre for Mental Health, 2012).

7.2 Initial contact

7.2.1 General principles and establishing rapport

Initial contact is particularly important, but it often occurs in less than ideal circumstances, such as in a busy emergency room. There may be concerns about the physical condition of the patient, and he or she may be mistrustful or even antagonistic towards others, including clinicians.

Considerable expertise and patience may be required to establish rapport. This may be achieved by emphasizing that the aim of the assessment is to try and understand what has happened and that time has been set aside to listen. Courtesy and respect for the individual is essential, and it is important to provide privacy. It is unrealistic to expect someone to divulge sensitive personal information unless confidentiality is assured. Of course, excellent communication skills will help the assessment and the clinician should be mindful of verbal and nonverbal cues. Patients often report that the most helpful aspect of a consultation is feeling listened to.

The individual should be given the opportunity to express his or her thoughts and feelings and allowed to discharge emotions. This 'catharsis' may put the person's suicidal intentions at least temporarily on hold. Open-ended questions are more likely to elicit useful information than closed questions. For some individuals, an enquiry about suicidal ideas may need a sensitive introduction before a more detailed exploration: for example, 'It sounds to me that you've been quite down recently ... Sometimes when people feel that bad they might have thoughts that they would like to go to sleep or not wake up ... or perhaps that they might even be better off dead. Have you ever felt like that?'.

While confidentiality is an important principle, in many situations the involvement of families is extremely important. Of course, patients need to consent to their information being shared in this way, but the danger is that professionals unnecessarily exclude family members from clinical management to the detriment of safety and quality of care (Department of Health Mental Health Equality and Disability Division, 2014).

7.2.2 Suicidal intent

Detailed enquiry about the circumstances of the suicidal behaviour is important in order to make a judgement about the degree of suicidal intent, from both the patient's and clinician's point of view. Sometimes reports of suicidal intent are unclear or minimized, and the context around the suicidal behaviour and the description of family members and significant others need to be considered. The following are important:

- What led up to the suicidal behaviour?
- How much planning had there been or was the behaviour relatively impulsive?
- What were the person's feelings about living and dying?
- What was the knowledge and expectation of the person about the potential lethality of their actions?
- Had there been any acts in anticipation of death, such as making a will or saying goodbye to family members?
- Had suicidal intent been expressed openly?
- Was the suicidal behaviour aimed at influencing others?
- Had the person acted to gain help during or after the attempt?
- Were precautions taken against discovery during the attempt?
- Did the behaviour occur in isolated circumstances, or where others could intervene?

Suicidal intent scales have been constructed using some of these factors, and elevated scores are associated with an increased risk of suicide in the long term (Beck et al., 1974; Stefansson et al., 2012). However, as with other measures of risk (see Chapter 8) they are of limited clinical utility in terms of prediction. Their use may ensure that clinicians address fully the individual components of suicidal intent. The value of assessing suicidal intent is not to try and predict the likelihood of future suicidal behaviour but to inform current treatment needs and the management plan.

7.2.3 Family history, past history, and bereavement by suicide

Family history of suicide, and a past history of suicidal behaviour (including its intent and lethality) increase suicide risk and it is important to enquire about these. Family history is not simply about a genetic risk but the increased risk associated with bereavement through suicide (Pitman et al., 2014). There is evidence that loss of a spouse, in particular, increases the risk of suicidal behaviour, but those who have lost other relatives, friends, or acquaintances are also vulnerable (see Chapter 13 for a fuller discussion). It is important that when a person reports having been bereaved by suicide that the professional explores the emotional impact of this loss (Pitman, 2018).

7.2.4 Means of suicide and role of the media

It is important to ask about the availability of means of suicide, and the focus of this enquiry may depend on the predominant method of suicide in that setting.

The availability of lethal medications or agricultural poisons should be addressed. If firearms are available, local laws about their possession may need to be invoked in regard to notifying firearms regulatory authorities. Care and sensitivity is required, and concern for safety should be emphasized.

Sometimes it is helpful to explore cognitive availability of methods and why particular methods were chosen. Did the person know someone who used a similar method? Was a novel method of self-injury identified from online sources? An enquiry about social media use might also be helpful, although of course it should be remembered that some people experience social media as beneficial to their mental well-being while for others it may be detrimental.

7.3 Mental state examination

An integral part of the assessment of someone with suicidal thoughts or behaviours is the mental state examination (analogous to the physical examination in general clinical practice). This occurs concurrently with the initial assessment of suicidal intent, and involves evaluating the person's appearance and behaviour in the interview, their speech pattern, their affective state, the presence of psychotic phenomena such as hallucinations and delusions, their cognitive state which may have been compromised by their suicidal behaviour, their capacity for introspection and insight, and their ability to form a therapeutic relationship.

Bearing in mind the importance of mood disorders in contributing to suicidal behaviour, it is sensible to ask specific questions about depression. The questions 'During the past month have you often been bothered by feeling down, depressed or hopeless?' and 'During the past month have you often been bothered by little interest or pleasure in doing things?', followed by 'Is this something with which you would like help?' have a high degree of sensitivity and specificity for delineating major depression (Arroll et al., 2005). But of course there are a number of ways of assessing depressive symptoms and disorders (National Collaborating Centre for Mental Health, 2009).

7.3.1 Clinical features which may be of concern

There are a number of concerning clinical features that may indicate a more urgent need for treatment. The expression of high suicidal intent, with severe depression, agitation, guilt, desperation, abandonment, humiliation, hopelessness, and a constriction of interest or self-absorption, should be taken particularly seriously (Hendin et al., 2007). So should 'malignant alienation'—a syndrome seen in those who have exhausted the patience and resources of friends and relatives and also of the helping professions, sometimes resulting in them being subjected to disparaging comments from others, including clinicians (Watts and Morgan, 1994). Other characteristics such as male gender, older age, choosing a high-lethality method, lack of social support, and ongoing substance misuse should also raise clinical concerns.

Although these factors are associated with suicide risk, the dilemma is that they lack predictive value for suicide. However, from a clinical perspective these should still be acted upon.

7.4 Hospitalization

Hospitalization may be necessary because of the physical effects of suicidal behaviour; if there are specific suicide plans, particularly with associated impulsivity; if an active psychotic illness is present; and if there is profound depression, hopelessness, and nihilism. The degree of social support a patient has may also influence the decision to hospitalize. But admission may not be suitable for all patients. In fact, for some it might be actively harmful. Recently, Large and colleagues have written about nosocomial suicide—the idea that it might actually be the toxic hospital environment that is directly responsible for some deaths (Large et al., 2014). On the other hand, Kapur et al. found, in a large observational study, that admission to a psychiatric bed may have saved lives in older people, men, and people with a past history of suicidal behaviour (Kapur et al., 2015). There does seem to be consensus that inpatient admission needs to be used for some patients and that wards should be as conducive to recovery as possible (Large and Kapur, 2018).

7.5 Compulsory treatment

The issue of compulsory treatment following self-harm (treating patients in the absence of informed consent or even contrary to their expressed views) is complex. Sometimes the clinician is working with an individual who sees no way out of their current difficulties, is ambivalent about future suicidal intent, and is suspicious or even hostile about the involvement of professionals. A full discussion of these issues is beyond the scope of this chapter, but further guidance is available both from the published literature, country-specific guidance, and guidance from medical defence organizations.

There are two aspects of treatment which need to be considered: treatment for the physical consequences of the suicide attempt and treatment for any underlying psychiatric disorder. They may be covered by different legislative frameworks (National Collaborating Centre for Mental Health, 2012). One issue is competence or whether patients have the 'capacity' to refuse treatment (defined broadly as being able to understand, retain, and weigh up information and communicate a decision). However, some clinicians argue that there is almost always sufficient doubt about capacity to initiate potentially lifesaving physical treatments after suicidal behaviour (Kapur, 2006).

Compulsory admission using appropriate mental health legislation may be required to reduce the risk to the patient or others. This management option is not one that should be taken lightly. It is a very significant decision to treat people against their wishes, as well as being potentially harmful and challenging. However, imposing constraints on a patient may buy time for the suicidal thoughts to dissipate. In these circumstances it is important to emphasize to the suicidal person, and his or her relatives or close others, that this management option is being considered because of concern for the person's welfare.

There are no RCTs to either support or refute the use of compulsory admission for some of those who have attempted suicide. It is a clinical decision which must sometimes be made with incomplete information. A UK case-control study of inpatient suicide found that those who had been detained for compulsory treatment during their last admission, or who had had enhanced levels of aftercare, were less likely to die by suicide (Hunt et al., 2007).

7.6 Benefits of comprehensive initial assessment

The importance of comprehensive initial assessment has been illustrated by studies which have followed up those who were not assessed adequately in emergency departments. One study found that patients who had self-harmed and left an accident and emergency department without a psychiatric assessment not only had a greater past history of self-harm but were also more likely to self-harm again in the subsequent year than a matched comparison group who had been assessed (Hickey et al., 2001). Findings from another study showed that patients who had deliberately self-poisoned and who had not received psychosocial assessment were more likely to poison themselves again (Kapur et al., 2002). Furthermore, this study suggested that only 12 patients needed to receive a psychosocial assessment to prevent one repetition of self-poisoning—a result which would have a marked effect on busy emergency departments. There have been similar findings in more recent studies, including those which have used robust statistical methods to adjust for confounding by indication—the fact that treatment allocation is not random and people with certain characteristics are more likely to receive an assessment (Carroll et al., 2016; Steeg et al., 2018).

The fact that something as simple as a clinical assessment may itself prevent repetition of suicidal behaviour is an important message for clinicians who sometimes view this patient group as difficult to help. How might such assessments work? It could be due to the therapeutic effect of the assessment itself, a feeling of being unburdened or listened to, or it may be that good assessments lead to more people being referred for appropriate aftercare (Kapur et al., 2013). Assessment may reduce the risk of future suicidal behavior by as much as 40%.

Box 7.1 Fundamentals of management

- Ensure safety
- If no psychiatric disorder:
  - active listening + follow-up
- If interpersonal/family issues:
  - active listening + problem-solving approach
  - consider referral to psychologist or social worker or other appropriate therapist for intervention
- If psychiatric disorder:
  - active listening + standard management for that disorder
  - appropriate psychotherapeutic support
  - consider psychiatric referral and psychotropic medication if indicated
- Consider offering psychological intervention in all cases

7.7 Need for subsequent management

During the initial assessment, the opportunity to express thoughts and feelings may in itself have been helpful (Sarfati et al., 2003). However, even if there is no psychiatric disorder, it is important to emphasize the goal of preventing further suicidal behaviour or self-harm. Follow-up could be offered to re-enforce alternative problem-solving methods. If psychiatric disorders are present, standard management practices should be followed (see Box 7.1).

Psychological interventions are known to be effective in preventing the repetition of suicidal behaviour. Specific options include cognitive behavioural, interpersonal, or problem-solving-based therapies. These are discussed further in Chapter 9. However, availability and routine access to these treatments remain an issue in many countries. Part of management strategies in many mental health services involves allocating treatment on the basis of presumed levels of risk of future suicidal behaviour. Although this seems to have face validity, it may not be the best approach We discuss this in detail in the next chapter.

7.8 Conclusion

The initial assessment of a person who presents with suicidal thoughts or behaviour can be one of the most challenging situations clinicians and other professionals encounter. Adhering to basic principles is important, as is specific inquiry about suicide. Often this initial contact is itself experienced as therapeutic, and it is crucial for engagement in further assessment and treatment. Figure 7.1 is an infographic summarizing the information in this chapter.

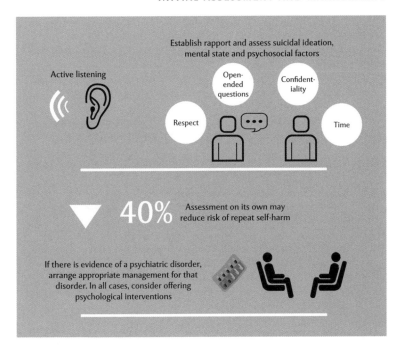

Fig 7.1 Initial assessment and management.
Courtesy of Dr Sarah Steeg.

REFERENCES

Arroll, B., Goodyear-Smith, F., Kerse, N., Fishman, T., and Gunn, J. (2005). Effect of the addition of a 'help' question to two screening questions on specificity for diagnosis of depression in general practice: diagnostic validity study. *BMJ* **331**(7521): 884.

Beck, A. T., Schuyler, D., and Herman, I. (1974). Development of suicidal intent scales. In *The Prediction of Suicide*, A. T. Beck, H. L. Resnik, and D. J. Lettieri (eds), pp. 45–56. Maryland: Charles Press Publishers.

Carroll, R., Metcalfe, C., Steeg, S., et al. (2016). Psychosocial assessment of self-harm patients and risk of repeat presentation: an instrumental variable analysis using time of hospital presentation. *PLoS One* **11**(2): e0149713.

Department of Health Mental Health Equality and Disability Division (2014). *Information Sharing and Suicide Prevention. Consensus Statement.* From https://assets.publishing. service.gov.uk/government/uploads/system/uploads/attachment_data/file/271792/ Consensus_statement_on_information_sharing.pdf

Goldney, R. D. (2005). Suicide prevention: a pragmatic review of recent studies. *Crisis* **26**(3): 128–40.

Gunnell, D. and Frankel, S. (1994). Prevention of suicide: aspirations and evidence. *BMJ* **308**(6938): 1227–33.

Hawton, K., Arensman, E., Townsend, E., et al. (1998). Deliberate self harm: systematic review of efficacy of psychosocial and pharmacological treatments in preventing repetition. *BMJ* **317**(7156): 441–7.

Hawton, K., Witt, K. G., Salisbury, T. L. T., et al. (2016). Psychosocial interventions following self-harm in adults: a systematic review and meta-analysis. *Lancet Psychiatry* **3**(8): 740–50.

Hendin, H., Maltsberger, J. T., and Szanto, K. (2007). The role of intense affective states in signaling a suicide crisis. *J Nerv Ment Dis* **195**(5): 363–8.

Hetrick, S. E., Robinson, J., Spittal, M. J., and Carter, G. (2016). Effective psychological and psychosocial approaches to reduce repetition of self-harm: a systematic review, meta-analysis and meta-regression. *BMJ Open* **6**(9): e011024.

Hickey, L., Hawton, K., Fagg, J., and Weitzel, H. (2001). Deliberate self-harm patients who leave the accident and emergency department without a psychiatric assessment: a neglected population at risk of suicide. *J Psychosom Res* **50**(2): 87–93.

Hunt, I. M., Kapur, N., Webb, R., et al. (2007). Suicide in current psychiatric in-patients: a case-control study The National Confidential Inquiry into Suicide and Homicide. *Psychol Med* **37**(6): 831–7.

Isacsson, G. and Rich, C. L. (2001). Management of patients who deliberately harm themselves. *BMJ* **322**(7280): 213–15.

Kapur, N. (2006). Self-harm in the general hospital. *Psychiatry* **5**(3): 76–80.

Kapur, N., Cooper, J., O'Connor, R. C., and Hawton, K. (2013). Non-suicidal self-injury v. attempted suicide: new diagnosis or false dichotomy? *Br J Psychiatry* **202**(5): 326–8.

Kapur, N., House, A., Dodgson, K., May, C., and Creed, F. (2002). Effect of general hospital management on repeat episodes of deliberate self poisoning: cohort study. *BMJ* **325**(7369): 866–7.

Kapur, N., Steeg, S., Turnbull, P., et al. (2015). Hospital management of suicidal behaviour and subsequent mortality: a prospective cohort study. *Lancet Psychiatry* **2**(9): 809–16.

Large, M., Ryan, C., Walsh, G., Stein-Parbury, J., and Patfield, M. (2014). Nosocomial suicide. *Australas Psychiatry* **22**(2): 118–21.

Large, M. M. and Kapur, N. (2018). Psychiatric hospitalisation and the risk of suicide. *Br J Psychiatry* **212**(5): 269–73.

Morriss, R., Kapur, N., and Byng, R. (2013). Assessing risk of suicide or self harm in adults. *BMJ* **347**: f4572.

National Collaborating Centre for Mental Health (2009). *Depression: The Treatment and Management of Depression in Adults*. Updated edition. From https://www.nice.org.uk/guidance/CG90

National Collaborating Centre for Mental Health (2012). *Self-Harm: Longer-Term Management*. Leicester: British Psychological Society.

National Collaborating Centre for Mental Health (2018). *Self-Harm and Suicide Prevention Competence Framework*. From https://www.ucl.ac.uk/pals/research/

clinical-educational-and-health-psychology/research-groups/core/competence-frameworks/self

Pitman, A. (2018). Addressing suicide risk in partners and relatives bereaved by suicide. *Br J Psychiatry* **212**(4): 197–8.

Pitman, A., Osborn, D., King, M., and Erlangsen, A. (2014). Effects of suicide bereavement on mental health and suicide risk. *Lancet Psychiatry* **1**(1): 86–94.

Sarfati, Y., Bouchaud, B., and Hardy-Bayle, M. C. (2003). Cathartic effect of suicide attempts not limited to depression: a short-term prospective study after deliberate self-poisoning. *Crisis* **24**(2): 73–8.

Steeg, S., Emsley, R., Carr, M., Cooper, J., and Kapur, N. (2018). Routine hospital management of self-harm and risk of further self-harm: propensity score analysis using record-based cohort data. *Psychol Med* **48**(2): 315–26.

Stefansson, J., Nordstrom, P., and Jokinen, J. (2012). Suicide Intent Scale in the prediction of suicide. *J Affect Disord* **136**(1–2): 167–71.

Watts, D. and Morgan, G. (1994). Malignant alienation. Dangers for patients who are hard to like. *Br J Psychiatry* **164**(1): 11–15.

CHAPTER 8

Risk assessment for suicide

KEY POINTS

- In mental health, 'risk' is often seen as negative, but it simply describes the likelihood of a particular event occurring.
- Clinical approaches to risk lack predictive validity, and risk scales perform no better.
- Novel risk markers or algorithms are unlikely to add much in the way of utility.
- Services should recognize the fallacy of risk prediction, and should instead focus on individual needs, comprehensive management plans, and ensuring care is as good as it possibly can be.

8.1 Introduction

The origins of the word 'risk' are uncertain. Some have suggested that it came into modern English from a Portuguese naval term for 'sailing into uncharted waters'; others say it derives from the Latin for 'cliff' or 'reef', or from the Ancient Greek for 'obstacles that were difficult to avoid in the sea'.

Probably the first scientific treatise on risk assessment in general was that of the sixteenth-century Italian physician and mathematician Girolamo Cardona (Bernstein, 1996). However, the concept does not appear to have been applied to suicide until 1954, when Rosen drew attention to the statistical limitation of the prediction of suicide on the basis of conventionally recognized risk factors. In the latter part of the twentieth century, a number of other studies demonstrated the same point (Goldney, 2000)—that it was not possible to predict suicide in an individual person.

Notwithstanding that limitation, in many parts of the world, risk assessment is a core component of mental health practice. It involves clinicians making judgements about the likelihood of future adverse outcomes. In epidemiological terms, risk refers simply to the likelihood of a particular event occurring, but in psychiatry, as in other areas, risk has taken on negative connotations. In clinical practice, we often talk about the risk of harm to self and others. This chapter will examine the role of risk assessment for suicide.

8.2 Basic concepts

Before a more detailed discussion, we should bear in mind two basic issues (Kapur, 2000). First, it is important to note that risk is continuous and not binary.

The high- and low-risk categorizations we often use in practice are arbitrary. Rather, there are degrees of risk. Second, risk is of course dynamic. It can change very quickly and certainly between one assessment and the next.

In many countries, risk assessment is a key part of the clinical care of people who are suicidal. The high-risk paradigm is a dominant one in that much of the effort in clinical practice is geared towards identifying people at highest risk (i.e. who most likely to go on to die by suicide) and then intervening with this group. However, there are difficulties with the high-risk approach and risk assessment more generally.

8.3 Clinical approaches to risk assessment

Clinical assessments of risk have been conceptualized as a 'balanced summary of prediction derived from knowledge of the individual, the present circumstances and what is known of the disorder from which he or she is suffering' or, alternatively, 'a prestigious synonym for anecdotal evidence' (Kapur, 2000).

Recent retrospective studies of risk prior to suicide have yielded some interesting findings. For example, data from the National Confidential Inquiry into Suicide in the UK—which collects data on all patients who die by suicide within 12 months of clinical contact—asked clinicians to rate the risk the last time they saw the patient. The results were surprising. In 80-90 per cent of cases, clinicians rated the immediate risk of suicide as low or absent (National Confidential Inquiry into Suicide and Safety in Mental Health, 2018a). Yet these patients all died. What might be the explanation for this low-risk paradox?

Of course this study involved retrospective global estimates of risk, and clinicians were not blind to the outcome. There may have been an element of defensive reporting. Risk is dynamic and it is also possible that the risk changed between the last assessment and death. However, half of patients were seen within seven days of dying.

A more detailed examination of the characteristics of individuals suggests they may not have been at quite as low a risk as the clinicians were reporting. Three quarters had a history of previous suicidal behaviour, nearly half had a history of alcohol misuse, and a third had a history of drug misuse. What this study perhaps demonstrates is a resetting of 'clinical risk barometers'. Because all the patients that clinical services see are essentially at 'high risk', clinical ratings of risk may get downgraded.

This was a retrospective study, but what does prospective research tell us? Studies of repetition of suicidal behaviour following clinical assessment show that those rated as at high risk by clinicians are at about twice the risk of repeating within one year of a self-harm episode (Kapur et al., 2005). However, in focusing our efforts on this high-risk group (even if we had interventions that were highly effective) we would miss the people in the low- and moderate-risk groups who repeated. Table 8.1 illustrates this. So an exclusive high-risk approach would result, at very best, in 95 repeat episodes being prevented. Importantly, though, because the lower-risk groups are much bigger than the high-risk group, 288 repeat

Table 8.1 Risk assessment and repetition of self-harm (Kapur et al., 2005)

Clinicians' rating of risk (N)	N (%) repeating self-harm within six months
Low (1721)	165 (9.6)
Moderate (1738)	288 (16.6)
High (369)	95 (25.7)

Adapted from *BMJ*, 330, Kapur N., Cooper J., Rodway C. et al., Predicting the risk of repetition after self harm: cohort study, pp. 394-395. Copyright © 2005, British Medical Journal Publishing Group. doi: https://doi.org/10.1136/bmj.38337.584225.82

episodes in the moderate-risk group and 165 in the low-risk group would be missed. This is an example of the population paradox. The results suggest that exclusively high-risk approaches to the prevention of future suicidal behaviour will not be effective (Kapur et al., 2015).

8.4 Risk scales

Actuaries are professionals who estimate risk and calculate insurance premiums. It has been argued that actuarial approaches to risk—risk-factor scales or tools—represent a more scientific, reliable, and valid means of assessment. In fact a number of systematic reviews have demonstrated that such scales may be of limited clinical utility (Chan et al., 2016; Quinlivan et al., 2016; Carter et al., 2017).

The predictive ability of scales can be highly variable but is limited because of the relatively low incidence of adverse outcomes. The positive predictive value of scales for predicting suicide after an episode of suicidal behaviour or self-harm is around 5 per cent (Carter et al., 2017). This means that for every one hundred people rated as at high risk, five go on to die by suicide. In other words, risk scales lack clinically useful predictive ability. What is even more important in practice is the large number of deaths that will get missed in the lower-risk groups—another example of the population paradox.

8.5 Clinical guidelines

The research findings have been reflected in the UK and Australian Clinical Guidelines which suggest that risk scales should not be used to predict future suicide or repetition of self-harm and should not be used to determine who is offered treatment and who should be discharged (National Collaborating Centre for Mental Health, 2011; Carter et al., 2016). Despite this, risk scales remain in widespread use. In one study of 31 hospitals in England, the vast majority of mental health staff used some form of risk-assessment tool or scale to assess their patients. Perhaps what was even more surprising was that in the majority of hospitals these tools had not been tested or validated and had simply been devised by the services themselves (Quinlivan et al., 2014). Another study of all 85 mental health services in the UK found that the number of different risk assessment tools in use was 156 (National Confidential Inquiry into Suicide and Safety in Mental Health, 2018b).

8.6 The best risk-assessment scales

Despite the well-documented problems with risk assessment, a question that is often asked is 'What is the best risk-assessment scale for suicidal behaviour?' A recent study tried to answer this question using a cohort design in a sample of people who presented to hospital following self-harm. The main outcome was repeat self-harm rather than suicide. Five risk scales with the most promising psychometric properties were compared against single items asking the clinician or the patient to rate, on a 10-point scale, how likely the latter was to repeat self-harm within six months (Quinlivan et al., 2017). The results were perhaps surprising. The best scales in this head-to-head cohort study of nearly five hundred people were the single-item ratings of risk by the clinician or the patient themselves. However, even these were not clinically useful. For example, the clinician scale missed nearly 20 per cent of people who went on to repeat, and nearly half of the people rated as at high risk by the scale did not repeat. A health economic modelling analysis of the same study suggested that if we used the clinician scale on a hundred people, 48 people would be rated at high risk, 25 high-risk people would not go on to repeat and would therefore receive unnecessary treatment, eight people who are actually high-risk would be missed, and only three people would be prevented from repeating self-harm (Quinlivan et al., 2019).

Qualitative data also illustrates the fact that clinicians and service users may not find risk-assessment scales particularly helpful. In some cases, a tick-box or checklist approach to assessment may be experienced as alienating and hamper therapeutic engagement (Stewart et al., 2018).

A recent large retrospective study (Steeg et al., 2018) suggested no difference in the accuracy of risk assessment when carried out by psychiatrists or mental health nurses and no important differences in accuracy by clinical subgroups. Scales do seem to perform even worse in patients seen by all services rather than those seen by just specialist mental health services. This may be because of the lower base rate of repetition (Steeg et al., 2018).

It should be acknowledged, however, that these studies are all based on observational data. There have been very few intervention studies. RCTs of risk assessment have mostly been restricted to the field of forensic psychiatry and violence risk assessments, and the findings have been variable.

8.7 Future developments in risk assessment

The development of novel risk measures is the subject of ongoing research. One approach is to use data-driven methods to derive the most important combination of risk factors in a development dataset and then test the instrument in a separate validation dataset. Examples of these empirically derived tools include the Manchester Self-Harm and ReACT rules and the RESH score. Although robustly developed, there is no good evidence that these tools are any more useful than older scales (Quinlivan et al., 2016).

A different approach is to use neurocognitive or psychological functioning as a marker of risk (Bolton et al., 2015). The advantage of some of these measures is that they can be used when people are unaware of their intent or not articulating it. Traits that may be predictive include deficits in attentional shifting, deficits in verbal fluency, and poor decision-making. Another novel method—the Implicit Association Test—measures the reaction time for people to respond to images (related to suicidal behaviour or neutral) (Nock et al., 2010). Shorter reaction times are thought to be associated with a greater propensity to suicidal behaviour. The predictive ability of the test may be improved when used in conjunction with other traditional risk factors.

Use of artificial intelligence or machine-learning methods for suicide risk have also been investigated (Walsh et al., 2017). Such approaches involve using computerized techniques to develop the best algorithms and statistical models for predicting suicide. Machine learning could help to inform precision or personalized medicine; that is, taking into account the individual genetic and environmental influences on a person's health in order to tailor treatments. A recent ambitious study showed the potential utility of this approach (Niculescu et al., 2017). There is certainly an argument that determining what works best for whom could be of greater benefit than adopting a 'one size fits all' approach. However, it has been pointed out that new methods of risk assessment would have to improve on existing ones by several orders of magnitude to be useful (Large et al., 2017). The performance of new tools would still be limited by the low (in population terms) base rate of suicide.

All these new developments are of interest but it is difficult to envisage how they might be usefully incorporated into clinical practice at this time. Perhaps a more fundamental research priority might be a large-cluster randomized trial of the effectiveness, including cost effectiveness, of conventional suicide risk assessment as an adjunct to usual care. To date, much of the evidence—or lack of evidence—for the utility of risk assessment has been from descriptive studies.

8.8 Conclusion: alternatives to a high-risk paradigm

If we accept that risk assessment and management according to a high-risk paradigm is not useful, then what should clinical services do instead? Perhaps the first thing that needs to happen is that clinicians should recognize the fallacy of risk assessment as risk prediction. It is simply impossible to predict which patients will go on to die by suicide and which will not. Risk assessment is often a process for assessing risks not for the individual patient, but for the organization or the individual clinician, and may often reflect defensive clinical practice.

Perhaps rather than a focus on risk, we should focus on individual patient needs. We should prioritize simple high-quality aspects of care. For example, in the UK, less than half of people who self-poison or injure themselves and then present to hospital are assessed by a mental health professional. Some descriptive data suggest that people who receive such an assessment are 40 per cent less likely to repeat self-harm (Kapur et al., 2013). We might also wish to make greater use of clinical guidelines and address the 'implementation gap' by making evidence-based treatments, such as cognitive behavioural therapy, more widely and easily available for people presenting with suicidal behaviour. Assessment should be individualized and always inform a management plan, rather than being an end in itself. Risk should never be a score or a red rating on a chart. Finally, based on evidence from other areas of population health (Kapur and House, 1998), there is a strong argument for adopting a population-based 'something for everyone' approach to suicide prevention. What this might mean in practice is that no patient with suicidal ideas or behaviours ever leaves mental health services empty-handed. Figure 8.1 is an infographic summarizing the information in this chapter.

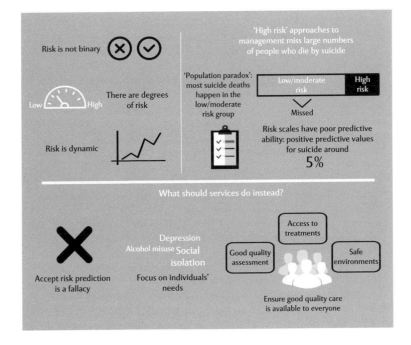

Fig 8.1 Suicide risk assessment.
Courtesy of Dr Sarah Steeg.

REFERENCES

Bernstein, P. L. (1996). *Against the Gods: The Remarkable Story of Risk*. New York: Wiley.

Bolton, J. M., Gunnell, D., and Turecki, G. (2015). Suicide risk assessment and intervention in people with mental illness. *BMJ* **351**: h4978.

Carter, G., Milner, A., McGill, K., Pirkis, J., Kapur, N., and Spittal, M. J. (2017). Predicting suicidal behaviours using clinical instruments: systematic review and meta-analysis of positive predictive values for risk scales. *Br J Psychiatry* **210**(6): 387–95.

Carter, G., Page, A., Large, M., et al. (2016). Royal Australian and New Zealand College of Psychiatrists clinical practice guideline for the management of deliberate self-harm. *Aust N Z J Psychiatry* **50**(10): 939–1000.

Chan, M. K., Bhatti, H., Meader, N., et al. (2016). Predicting suicide following self-harm: systematic review of risk factors and risk scales. *Br J Psychiatry* **209**(4): 277–83.

Goldney, R. (2000). Prediction of suicide and attempted suicide. In *The International Handbook of Suicide and Attempted Suicide*, K. Hawton and K. van Heeringen (eds), pp. 585–95. Chichester: John Wiley.

Kapur, N. (2000). Evaluating risks. *Adv Psychiatr Treat* **6**(6): 399–406.

Kapur, N., Cooper, J., Rodway, C., Kelly, J., Guthrie, E., and Mackway-Jones, K. (2005). Predicting the risk of repetition after self harm: cohort study. *BMJ* **330**(7488): 394–5.

Kapur, N. and House. A. (1998). Against a high-risk strategy in the prevention of suicide. *Psychiatr Bull* **22**(9): 534–6.

Kapur, N., Steeg, S., Turnbull, P., et al. (2015). Hospital management of suicidal behaviour and subsequent mortality: a prospective cohort study. *Lancet Psychiatry* **2**(9): 809–16.

Kapur, N., Steeg, S., Webb, R., et al. (2013). Does clinical management improve outcomes following self-harm? Results from the multicentre study of self-harm in England. *PLoS One* **8**(8): e70434.

Large, M. M., Ryan, C. J., Carter, G., and Kapur, N. (2017). Can we usefully stratify patients according to suicide risk? *BMJ* **359**: j4627.

National Collaborating Centre for Mental Health (2011). *Self-Harm: Longer-Term Management*. NICE Clinical Guideline 133. Manchester: National Institute for Health and Care Excellence.

Niculescu, A. B., Le-Niculescu, H., Levey, D. F., et al. (2017). Precision medicine for suicidality: from universality to subtypes and personalization. *Mol Psychiatry* **22**(9): 1250–73.

The National Confidential Inquiry into Suicide and Safety in Mental Health (NCISH) (2018a). Annual Report: England, Northern Ireland, Scotland, Wales. October 2018. University of Manchester.

The National Confidential Inquiry into Suicide and Safety in Mental Health (NCISH) (2018b). *The assessment of clinical risk in mental health services*. Manchester: The University of Manchester, 2018.

Nock, M. K., Park, J. M., Finn, C. T., Deliberto, T. L., Dour, H. J., and Banaji, M. R. (2010). Measuring the suicidal mind: implicit cognition predicts suicidal behavior. *Psychol Sci* **21**(4): 511–17.

Quinlivan, L., Cooper, J., Davies, L., Hawton, K., Gunnell, D., and Kapur, N. (2016). Which are the most useful scales for predicting repeat self-harm? A systematic review evaluating risk scales using measures of diagnostic accuracy. *BMJ Open* 6(2).

Quinlivan, L., Cooper, J., Meehan, D., et al. (2017). Predictive accuracy of risk scales following self-harm: multicentre, prospective cohort study. *Br J Psychiatry* 210(6): 429–36.

Quinlivan, L., Cooper, J., Steeg, S., et al. (2014). Scales for predicting risk following self-harm: an observational study in 32 hospitals in England. *BMJ Open* 4(5): e004732.

Quinlivan, L., Steeg, S., Elvidge, J., et al. (2019). Risk assessment scales to predict risk of hospital treated repeat self-harm: a cost-effectiveness modelling analysis. *J Affect Disord* 249: 208–15. https://doi.org/10.1016/j.jad.2019.02.036

Steeg, S., Quinlivan, L., Nowland, R., et al. (2018). Accuracy of risk scales for predicting repeat self-harm and suicide: a multicentre, population-level cohort study using routine clinical data. *BMC Psychiatry* 18(1): 113.

Stewart, A., Hughes, N. D., Simkin, S., et al. (2018). Navigating an unfamiliar world: how parents of young people who self-harm experience support and treatment. *Child Adolesc Ment Health* 23(2): 78–84.

Walsh, C. G., Ribeiro, J. D., and Franklin, J. C. (2017). Predicting risk of suicide attempts over time through machine learning. *Clin Psychol Sci* 5(3): 457–69.

CHAPTER 9

Psychological and other non-pharmacological approaches

> **KEY POINTS**
>
> - All people who present with suicidal thoughts and behaviours warrant intervention, the nature and intensity of which depend on their individual needs.
> - Psychological treatments which may help include cognitive behavioural therapy (CBT), interpersonal therapy (IPT), problem-solving therapy, and mindfulness-based cognitive behavioural therapy (MCBT).
> - Dialectical behaviour therapy is specifically designed for those with a diagnosis of borderline personality disorder.
> - Therapies should probably be time limited in most cases but there is a balance between avoiding therapeutic dependence and being perceived as rejecting.
> - Broader non-pharmacological approaches include crisis centres, volunteer organizations, brief-contact interventions (e.g.postcards or telephone calls), and safety plans. These need further investigation in research studies.

9.1 General approach

Many of those with suicidal thoughts or who have harmed themselves may benefit from some form of emotional support or psychological intervention as part of a needs-based approach to management. Two major systematic reviews have explored this issue recently. Hawton and colleagues found a reduction in the rate of repetition in patients who had received cognitive behavioural-type therapy versus treatment as usual (OR 0.70 (95%CI 0.55–0.88)) (Hawton et al., 2016). Hetrick et al. reported a 16 per cent reduction in the risk of repetition for people provided with psychosocial intervention versus usual care, with 33 people needing to be treated to prevent one repeat episode (Hetrick et al., 2016). Meta-regression showed that the type of intervention did not modify the treatment effects. In other words there was no good evidence that any one therapeutic approach was better than any other.

In practice, clinicians often adopt a practical problem-solving approach to help a person develop alternative ways of coping in the future. If a psychiatric disorder is present, standard evidence-based treatments should be followed (National Collaborating Centre for Mental Health, 2012). If medication is indicated, concurrent emotional support should still be offered as well. The nature of this will depend on the age of the patient, and should involve parents of children and adolescents, or other family members or friends of adults. Online resources may be helpful: for example, information for the parents of children who self-harm is available via the Health Talk website in the UK (Healthtalk. org, 2014). Interventions should be accessible and tailored appropriately to groups who might have specific needs such as black and ethnic minority and LGBT groups.

9.2 Psychological treatments

Studies have demonstrated the effectiveness of cognitive behavioural therapy (CBT) and interpersonal therapy (IPT) after self-harm in reducing depression, suicidal ideation, and repeat episodes (Stoffers et al., 2012; Hawton et al., 2016; Hetrick et al., 2016). Problem-solving and behavioural therapies have also been used. Mindfulness-based cognitive behavioural therapy (MCBT) has shown some promise in reducing the likelihood of re-emergence of suicidal ideation in those who have experienced it in the past (Williams et al., 2006). Patients in all of these studies did not have psychotic illnesses, but there is no reason to assume that these individuals would not benefit from provision of additional psychotherapies (see Box 9.1).

9.2.1 Cognitive behavioural therapy

The aim of CBT is to identify inaccuracies in an individual's thoughts about themselves and their wider world, to modify these, and to guide the person towards mastery of their thoughts and actions. This can then minimize the likelihood of further suicidal behaviour (Berk et al., 2004; Slee et al., 2007; Stoffers et al., 2012).

CBT is based on the observation that those with suicidal thoughts or behaviours may sometimes see themselves as inadequate and unworthy. They might view any interaction with others as demanding and tend to downplay successful experiences. They typically have negative expectations of the future, anticipating that any initiatives are doomed from the start. Therapy is designed to counteract these inaccuracies of cognition, and involves both cognitive and behavioural techniques.

Patients are asked to define specific thoughts that are plausible to them but which can, in fact, be self-defeating. The therapist then assists the patient in what is, in essence, a detailed examination of the statement, looking at evidence which supports and contradicts it. This is done in a non-judgemental manner. The inaccuracy of the thought is explored and the patient is invited to generate alternative explanations. This is an important part of identifying maladaptive assumptions, as it provides the patient with alternative modes of thinking that may be less negative. To illustrate this point, people who present with suicidal thoughts may believe they are failures in all aspects of their lives. By asking them to step outside themselves and view themselves as others would, areas of competence (such as the ability to work, play sport, or raise children) may be identified. The original assumption can start to be seen as inaccurate. The therapist can then explore how it is these successes have occurred. Patients may subsequently be able to acknowledge that they must have had positive attributes and skills in order to have contributed to that successful outcome.

The behavioural component of CBT is similar in principle and is based on scheduling activities that can actually be mastered by the patient, and which provide alternatives to suicidal behaviour. Ultimate goals of treatment that might initially be regarded as very difficult, or even impossible, are identified and then broken down into a series of graded tasks or steps. The successful completion of each task provides immediate confirmation to the patient of their own capability. Such activities can initially take the form of imagined 'cognitive rehearsal' or role play. However, it is also important that real-life tasks are carried out fairly promptly, in order to provide reassurance of the patient's 'mastery'.

An important aspect of CBT is to have an agenda for each session, with a list of priorities that can be achieved. It is also helpful to have 'homework', for which unhelpful thoughts are recorded along with alternative hypotheses. Some patients may need to focus upon much smaller steps than others, and it is important that continuous and positive feedback on achievements be given at each session. It is helpful to maintain a problem-orientated stance and keep patients focused on concrete, achievable goals. This will help to reinforce positive self-esteem and may make suicidal behaviour less likely.

9.2.2 Interpersonal therapy and psychodynamic interpersonal therapy

Interpersonal therapy (IPT) was developed in the 1970s to treat depression, and it aims to elicit, clarify, and place into perspective those feelings that have arisen from interaction with others in the social environment (Weissman et al., 2007). It can be useful because suicidal behaviour invariably occurs in a psychosocial and interpersonal context.

The focus is on current problems, anxieties, and frustrations, with an effort being made to define problems in 'here and now' terms. Loss and threatened loss are important, as are ambivalent feelings about them. Eliciting these mixed feelings about loss may be particularly helpful as one of the classic formulations of suicidal behaviour is that the person is unable to come to terms with angry feelings regarding losses, and there is fear of guilt about those emotions. Instead, these angry feelings are turned inwards against the self, thereby precipitating the suicidal behaviour. Therapists need to be aware of such feelings and encourage their expression. Sometimes losses may not be readily apparent, and a careful history elucidating relationships with parents, siblings, children, and significant others is necessary. This is facilitated by an interpersonal inventory, which provides struc-ture to the therapy sessions.

It is important to remember that suicidal behaviour has a large interpersonal/communication component, and it often occurs in the context of interpersonal rejection. While IPT appears a logical approach, there is no definitive evidence of its effectiveness in preventing suicidal behaviour, although it does prevent relapse in those who have been depressed (Frank et al., 2007).

Psychodyanamic interpersonal therapy (PIT) involves using the patient–therapist relationship to identify and help resolve interpersonal difficulties which cause or exacerbate psychological distress. The model (sometimes referred to as the conversational model) was developed by Hobson, and in one random-ized trial, the intervention was associated with fewer suicidal ideas, fewer de-pressive symptoms, and a reduction in self-reported repeat self-harm (Guthrie et al., 2001).

9.2.3 Problem-solving therapy

Those who attempt suicide may have poorer 'problem-solving' ability, and this persists despite changes in mood (Pollock and Williams, 2004). Problem-solving therapy is partly based on the premise that symptoms are related to everyday problems which, if resolved, will lead to alleviation of symptoms (Reinecke, 2006). However, other clinicians highlight enduring poor problem-solving ability as a core deficit and adopt a more skills- based stance. That is, the main aim of therapy is to improve problem-solving skills rather than to resolve problems per se.

Initially, the patient describes their symptoms and problems, and these are linked where possible. This provides a rationale for addressing the problem. Major problems can be split into their components, and potential solutions can be generated by the patient and therapist. The preferred solution can then be ar-rived at by discussion of the pros and cons of each course of action. The solution can then be practised in imagination and role play. The individual is then encour-aged to try out the new problem-solving techniques in his or her everyday life and personal relationships.

Review of progress is essential, as is encouragement to persist. Sometimes it might be necessary to modify the preferred problem-solving technique. Although the therapy shows promise (Hetrick et al., 2016), a randomized trial from New Zealand of a package of care including problem-solving therapy (as well as regular contact through postcards) showed little difference in outcomes compared with usual care. The study authors highlighted some possible reasons for the lack of an effect, including difficulties accessing the treatment and a relatively low dose of therapy (Hatcher et al., 2011).

9.2.4 Mindfulness-based cognitive behavioural therapy

Mindfulness-based cognitive behavioural therapy (MBCT) uses aspects of CBT with meditation techniques from Buddhism (Williams et al., 2006). It is intensive and requires considerable commitment. In some models there are seven, weekly, two-hour classes, and an all-day practice between the sixth and seventh classes, as well as individual daily practice. Various aspects of bodily experience are focused on, so that participants become aware of small sensations that previously might have passed unnoticed. The role of negative thoughts, ruminations, and emotions in perpetuating distress is addressed, but more so that they can be accepted as simply thoughts and emotions, and not necessarily important or reflections of reality. While this approach shows promise, it is important to note that it may be less useful as an acute treatment, but more useful as a technique to prevent recurrence of suicidal behaviour. It has shown some benefit in reducing suicidal ideation in people who are depressed (Forkmann et al., 2014).

9.2.5 Dialectical behaviour therapy

Dialectical behaviour therapy (DBT) (Linehan et al., 1991) involves cognitive, behavioural, and supportive techniques, and is specifically designed for those with borderline personality disorder. A meta-analysis of a number of studies has demonstrated a reduction in self-harm and improvement in general functioning (Stoffers et al., 2012). However, the recent review by Hawton and colleagues did not find a reduction in the number of individuals repeating self-harm in those receiving DBT, but there was a reduction in the overall number of self-harm episodes (Hawton et al., 2016).

The DBT model of treatment is demanding on both patient and therapist. It addresses:

- The patient's behavioural capabilities
- Motivation for desirable behaviours
- The structure of the treatment environment to reinforce adaptive behaviour
- The generalizability of gains
- The therapist's capabilities and motivation.

The full model is intensive, with one hour's weekly individual psychotherapy, two and a half hours per week of group skills training, telephone consultations on an 'as needed' basis, and weekly therapist team meetings as well.

Variations on this rigorous DBT approach have been used in some other studies. For example, a large multi-centre randomized trial used manual assisted cognitive behavioural therapy, which incorporated DBT concepts. However, this study found no difference in the repetition of self-harm between the experimental and treatment-as-usual groups (Tyrer et al., 2003). It should be noted that participants were not selected on the basis of their clinical diagnosis as is the case for DBT.

> **Box 9.1** Individual psychotherapies
>
> - All people presenting with suicidal thoughts or behaviours should be offered emotional support.
> - Psychotherapies with evidence for effectiveness include:
>   - cognitive behavioural therapy
>   - interpersonal therapy/psychodynamic interpersonal therapy
>   - problem-solving therapy
>   - mindfulness-based cognitive behavioural therapy.
> - Dialectical behaviour therapy is specific for those with borderline personality disorder.

9.2.6 Completing the course of therapy

Whichever therapy is undertaken (see Box 9.1 for a summary), there may be a fine line between avoiding therapeutic dependence in patients and appearing to reject those who are in distress. The fostering of independence can be facilitated by the therapist making it clear to the patient that his or her involvement will be time-limited and then, at the end of that time (if appropriate), expressing confidence in the person's ability to cope in the future.

While a circumscribed time-limited course of therapy is probably best for most patients, some (such as young adults with few family and social supports, those with borderline personality diorder, and patients with chronic psychiatric illness) may require longer-term psychotherapeutic contact. In these instances there may also be encouragement for a degree of self-management, with appropriate professional support, as well as making contingency plans for crises.

9.3 Broader non-pharmacological approaches

9.3.1 Crisis centres and the role of volunteers

The first telephone crisis centres intended to prevent suicide were established in the USA in the early twentieth century. However, the main impetus for their further development was provided by Chad Varah, a clergyman, who founded the Samaritans in England in 1953. Since then there have been similar initiatives in many countries, usually under the auspices of volunteer organizations such as the Samaritans, the International Federation of Telephone Emergency Services (IFOTES), and Lifeline (Scott, 1996). There are major methodological challenges in demonstrating their effectiveness, but one review of 14 studies concluded that overall there was an impact on suicidal behaviour in those areas which had such centres (Lester, 1997). Furthermore, significant decreases in measures of suicidality between the beginning and end of telephone counselling sessions have been reported (Gould et al., 2007).

The effective components of crisis centres may be that they are readily accessible; they are available 24 hours a day; and they are acceptable to some who may not access alternative services or who prefer their anonymity. The notion of non-judgemental acceptance is extended to face-to-face contact in some volunteer organizations, where the principles of 'befriending' apply. This may involve regular contact of up to once a week, talking, listening, and 'being there' for practical issues. One review suggests this approach is effective in reducing depressive symptoms and emotional distress (Mead et al., 2010).

'Befriending' was used in a project in Sri Lanka, initiated by Sumithrayo, a volunteer organization dedicated to suicide prevention (Maracek and Ratnayeke, 2000). In response to suicidal behaviour in rural areas, befriending support was offered to one village, with another village used as a comparison. The village which received the intervention had had 13 suicide deaths and 18 other episodes of self-harm in the six years before the programme, but there were no episodes of suicidal behaviour in the subsequent four and a half years. That contrasted with the comparison village, which previously had 16 suicide deaths and 25 other episodes of self-harm, and which had a further three suicide deaths and 10 other episodes of self-harm in the next two years. Following this, the investigators extended the programme to that village.

Robust evaluations of helplines and similar initiatives are difficult, and many studies restrict themselves to investigating user acceptability, access, or process rather than outcomes (Zalsman et al., 2016). Helplines and similar interventions are now being provided through a variety of innovative physical and digital means (e.g. text or SMS, online chat) (Mokkenstorm et al., 2017). These initiatives need to be investigated in future research studies.

9.3.2 Other approaches

9.3.2.1 Postcards and brief-contact interventions

A deceptively simple form of ongoing written contact with people who had attempted suicide in the USA resulted in a significant reduction in suicide for the duration of the contact (Motto and Bostrom, 2001). Those who had attempted suicide were contacted one month after their suicide attempt, and those who had not pursued further treatment were randomly assigned to contact and no-contact groups. The contact group received correspondence each month for four months, then every two months for eight months, and then every three months for a further four years—a total of five years and 24 contacts per person. The contact usually involved a short letter, but sometimes a phone call, and each letter was worded slightly differently and included responses if previous contact had been reciprocated. The letters simply noted that it was some time since the person had been at the hospital, that it was hoped all was well, and that they could make contact if they wished. Over a five-year period there were fewer deaths by suicide in those who had had contact when compared with the no-contact group. However, longer-term follow-up indicated that the differences reduced over time and the suicide rates were identical after 14 years.

Since that study was undertaken, similar interventions have been tested in the UK, Australia, New Zealand, and Iran, with more equivocal results. The interventions may have more impact on the frequency of repetition than the likelihood that someone will repeat. They may also have more impact on women and people with a past history of self-harm episodes. The importance of the context in which messages and postcards are provided is important. It is possible they have more effect in settings where little is available in terms of usual treatment (Kapur et al., 2010). They may also have side effects: one very small pilot study suggested people who received contact were more likely to repeat than those who did not (Kapur et al., 2013). Some people may want to forget about an isolated episode of suicidal behaviour rather than be reminded of it through regular postcards (Goldney et al., 2009). Nevertheless, such approaches show some promise and could be refined to determine what specific follow-up approach may be suitable for which persons and in which setting (Kapur et al., 2010; Cooper et al., 2011; Milner et al., 2016).

9.3.2.2 Safety planning

'Safety plans' are in widespread use in many mental health services but the evidence base supporting their use is limited. A safety plan is a collaboratively developed list of practical, personalized coping skills and strategies for the patient to use when suicide risk is elevated (Stanley and Brown, 2012): for example, recognizing early warning signs, what action to take, or who to contact. A number of apps offer online safety planning. This is an area of ongoing research.

A recent large prospective non-randomized comparison of safety planning and telephone contact versus usual treatment in over 1,600 attenders to emergency departments in the USA showed an almost halving in the risk of repetition of suicidal behaviour in the intervention versus control group at six months (3 per cent versus 5.3 per cent), with a doubling in the likelihood of attending at least one mental health outpatient appointment (Stanley et al., 2018). This is a potentially important study, but it should be noted that it was carried out in Veterans Health Administration hospitals and the overall rate of repetition was low compared to clinical samples internationally (Carroll et al., 2014). This may raise some questions about the extent to which the findings are generalizable. Further research into safety planning is needed.

9.4 Conclusion—common therapeutic components

In general, there are common elements in many non-pharmacological approaches, and these are summarized in Box 9.2. People are assessed and treated

---

Box 9.2 Common therapeutic components

- A respectful approach
- A non-judgemental attitude
- Embody warmth, genuineness, and empathy
- Provide a sense of 'connectedness to others'.

---

with respect and seriousness; the individual face-to-face interventions are not open-ended, but structured and with agreed objectives, sometimes using a manual-based approach. Crisis centres and volunteers provide a readily accessible and non-judgemental point of contact, which can allow time for the crisis to dissipate. These interventions often involve a sense of reaching out and offering support. Indeed, the title of one research study investigating the general issue was: 'Well it's like someone at the other end cares about you' (Cooper et al., 2011).

The overall therapeutic approach should embrace the concepts of warmth, genuineness, and empathy, which have been shown to be of benefit in effective psychotherapy (Truax et al., 1971) and may enhance a sense of 'connectedness to others' (Frank, 1971). Figure 9.1 is an infographic summarizing the information in this chapter.

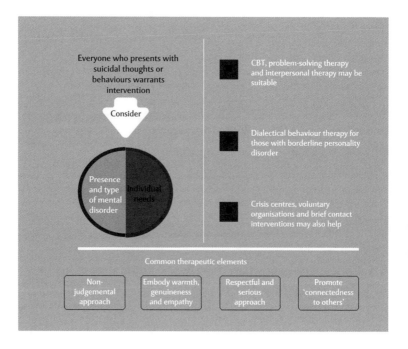

Fig 9.1 Psychological and other non-pharmacological interventions for suicide prevention.

Courtesy of Dr Sarah Steeg.

REFERENCES

Berk, M. S., Henriques, G. R., Warman, D. M., Brown, G. K., and Beck, A. T. (2004). A cognitive therapy intervention for suicide attempters: an overview of the treatment and case examples. *Cogn Behav Pract* **11**(3): 265–77.

Carroll, R., Metcalfe, C., and Gunnell, D. (2014). Hospital presenting self-harm and risk of fatal and non-fatal repetition: systematic review and meta-analysis. *PLoS One* **9**(2): e89944.

Cooper, J., Hunter, C., Owen-Smith, A., et al. (2011). "Well it's like someone at the other end cares about you." A qualitative study exploring the views of users and providers of care of contact-based interventions following self-harm. *Gen Hosp Psychiatry* **33**(2): 166–76.

Forkmann, T., Wichers, M., Geschwind, N., et al. (2014). Effects of mindfulness-based cognitive therapy on self-reported suicidal ideation: results from a randomised controlled trial in patients with residual depressive symptoms. *Compr Psychiatry* **55**(8): 1883–90.

Frank, E., Kupfer, D. J., Buysse, D. J., et al. (2007). Randomized trial of weekly, twice-monthly, and monthly interpersonal psychotherapy as maintenance treatment for women with recurrent depression. *Am J Psychiatry* **164**(5): 761–7.

Frank, J. D. (1971). Eleventh Emil A. Gutheil memorial conference. Therapeutic factors in psychotherapy. *Am J Psychother* **25**(3): 350–61.

Goldney, R. D., Winefield, A. H., Winefield, H. R., and Saebel, J. (2009). The benefit of forgetting suicidal ideation. *Suicide Life Threat Behav* **39**(1): 33–7.

Gould, M. S., Kalafat, J., Harrismunfakh, J. L., and Kleinman, M. (2007). An evaluation of crisis hotline outcomes. Part 2: Suicidal callers. *Suicide Life Threat Behav* **37**(3): 338–52.

Guthrie, E., Kapur, N., Mackway-Jones, K., et al. (2001). Randomised controlled trial of brief psychological intervention after deliberate self poisoning. *BMJ* **323**(7305): 135–8.

Hatcher, S., Sharon, C., Parag, V., and Collins, N. (2011). Problem-solving therapy for people who present to hospital with self-harm: Zelen randomised controlled trial. *Br J Psychiatry* **199**(4): 310–16.

Hawton, K., Witt, K. G., Salisbury, T. L. T., et al. (2016). Psychosocial interventions following self-harm in adults: a systematic review and meta-analysis. *Lancet Psychiatry* **3**(8): 740–50.

Healthtalk.org (2014). *Self-Harm: Parents' Experiences*. From http://www.healthtalk.org/peoples-experiences/mental-health/self-harm-parents-experiences/topics

Hetrick, S. E., J. Robinson, M. J. Spittal and G. Carter (2016). 'Effective psychological and psychosocial approaches to reduce repetition of self-harm: a systematic review, meta-analysis and meta-regression'. *BMJ Open* **6**(9): e011024.

Kapur, N., Cooper, J., Bennewith, O., Gunnell, D., and Hawton, K. (2010). Postcards, green cards and telephone calls: therapeutic contact with individuals following self-harm. *Br J Psychiatry* **197**(1): 5–7.

Kapur, N., Cooper, J., O'Connor, R. C., and Hawton, K. (2013). Non-suicidal self-injury v. attempted suicide: new diagnosis or false dichotomy? *Br J Psychiatry* **202**(5): 326–8.

Lester, D. (1997). The effectiveness of suicide prevention centers: a review. *Suicide Life Threat Behav* **27**(3): 304–10.

Linehan, M. M., Armstrong, H. E., Suarez, A., Allmon, D., and Heard, H. L. (1991). Cognitive-behavioral treatment of chronically parasuicidal borderline patients. *Arch Gen Psychiatry* **48**(12): 1060–4.

Maracek, J. and Ratnayeke, L. (2000). Suicide in rural Sri Lanka: assessing a prevention programme. In *Suicide Risk and Protective Factors in the New Millenium*, O. T. Grad (ed.), pp. 215–19. Ljubljana: Cankarjev dom.

Mead, N., Lester, H., Chew-Graham, C., Gask, L., and Bower, P. (2010). Effects of befriending on depressive symptoms and distress: systematic review and meta-analysis. *Br J Psychiatry* **196**(2): 96–101.

Milner, A., Spittal, M. J., Kapur, N., Witt, K., Pirkis, J., and Carter, G. (2016). Mechanisms of brief contact interventions in clinical populations: a systematic review. *BMC Psychiatry* **16**: 194.

Mokkenstorm, J. K., Eikelenboom, M., Huisman, A., et al. (2017). Evaluation of the 113 online suicide prevention crisis chat service: outcomes, helper behaviors and comparison to telephone hotlines. *Suicide Life Threat Behav* **47**(3): 282–96.

Motto, J. A. and Bostrom, A. G. (2001). A randomized controlled trial of postcrisis suicide prevention. *Psychiatr Serv* **52**(6): 828–33.

National Collaborating Centre for Mental Health (2012). *Self-Harm: Longer-Term Management*. Leicester: British Psychological Society.

Pollock, L. R. and Williams, J. M. (2004). Problem-solving in suicide attempters. *Psychol Med* **34**(1): 163–7.

Reinecke, M. A. (2006). Problem solving: a conceptual approach to suicidality and psychotherapy. In *Cognition and Suicide: Theory, Research and Therapy*, T. Ellis (ed.), pp. 237–60. Washington DC: American Psychological Association.

Scott, V. (1996). Reaching the suicidal: the volunteer's role in preventing suicide—a column from Befrienders International. *Crisis* **17**(3): 102–4.

Slee, N., Arensman, E., Garnefski, N., and Spinhoven, P. (2007). Cognitive-behavioral therapy for deliberate self-harm. *Crisis* **28**(4): 175–82.

Stanley, B. and Brown, G. K. (2012). Safety planning intervention: a brief intervention to mitigate suicide risk. *Cogn Behav Pract* **19**(2): 256–64.

Stanley, B., Brown, G. K., Brenner, L. A., et al. (2018). Comparison of the safety planning intervention with follow-up vs usual care of suicidal patients treated in the emergency department. *JAMA Psychiatry* **75**(9): 894–900.

Stoffers, J. M., Vollm, B. A., Rucker, G., Timmer, A., Huband, N., and , Lieb, K. (2012). Psychological therapies for people with borderline personality disorder. *Cochrane Database Syst Rev*(8): CD005652.

Truax, C. B., Wittmer, J., and Wargo, D. G. (1971). Effects of the therapeutic conditions of accurate empathy, non-possessive warmth, and genuineness on hospitalized mental patients during group therapy. *J Clin Psychol* **27**(1): 137–42.

Tyrer, P., Thompson, S., Schmidt, U., et al. (2003). Randomized controlled trial of brief cognitive behaviour therapy versus treatment as usual in recurrent deliberate self-harm: the POPMACT study. *Psychol Med* **33**(6): 969–76.

Weissman, M. M., Markowitz, J. C., and Klerman, G. L. (2007). *Clinician's Quick Guide to Interpersonal Psychotherapy*. New York: Oxford University Press.

Williams, J. M., Duggan, D. S., Crane, C., and Fennell, M. J. (2006). Mindfulness-based cognitive therapy for prevention of recurrence of suicidal behavior. *J Clin Psychol* **62**(2): 201–10.

Zalsman, G., Hawton, K., Wasserman, D., et al. (2016). Suicide prevention strategies revisited: 10-year systematic review. *Lancet Psychiatry* **3**(7): 646–59.

CHAPTER 10

Pharmacological approaches

> **KEY POINTS**
>
> - The use of medication in those who present with suicidal thoughts or behaviours has been controversial.
> - If there is a psychiatric disorder for which there is evidence of effective pharmacological treatment, then that treatment should be offered.
> - There is research evidence to suggest that antidepressants, mood stabilizers, and antipsychotic medications can be effective in reducing suicidality.
> - Ketamine, a short-acting anaesthetic and NMDA receptor antagonist, is potentially helpful and is the subject of much research.

10.1 Concerns about medication

There are some concerns about the role of psychotropic medication in the management of those who present with suicidal thoughts or behaviours. Indeed, the question has even been posed as to whether such medication should be prescribed for this group at all. Even stronger views have been expressed about the pharmacological treatment of young people.

The reservations about drug treatment centre around a number of issues. For example, the medicalization of 'normal' interpersonal and family problems; the risk of medication being used in overdose; and reports that antidepressants could precipitate suicidal behaviour, particularly in young people. These concerns are understandable but medication can have an important role as part of a treatment plan. Medication should only be prescribed if clinically indicated for a specific underlying psychiatric disorder. Suicidal behaviour per se is not an indication. Of course there is always some risk of further suicidal behaviour, and the safest (least toxic) medications should be prescribed. With regard to the possibility of antidepressants precipitating suicidal behaviour, there are certainly some concerns in young people, but the balance of harm and benefit is in favour of treatment in adults. Antidepressants may also sometimes be the right therapeutic option in young people.

In general, if suicidal behaviour is associated with a psychiatric disorder for which there is an effective evidence-based pharmacological treatment, then that treatment should be offered. Naturally this should be provided with therapeutic support and monitoring of the medication during follow-up consultations. There should be due regard for adherence and potential side effects, as well as psychological interventions as appropriate.

10.2 Potential benefits of pharmacotherapy

Historically, it has been assumed that by treating the mental disorders associated with suicidal behaviours, those behaviours will be reduced. In the UK during the early 1970s it was suggested that as many as a fifth of people who died by suicide might have benefitted from lithium because of their recurrent affective disorders (Barraclough, 1972). Swiss research several decades later, in a sample of patients hospitalized for mood disorders and followed up over many years, reported that a significantly higher proportion of those who survived had been receiving psychotropic drugs, including lithium, than those who had died (Angst et al., 2002). A study from New York found that 16.4 per cent of 1,635 people who had died by suicide were on psychotropic medication. The authors suggested that it was unexpected that there had not been greater prescription of standard psychotropic drugs prior to death, bearing in mind the known association between psychiatric disorders and suicide (Marzuk et al., 1995). Similar findings were later reported from Finland, Sweden, and Switzerland. Additional findings from more specific studies involving antidepressant, mood stabilizer, and antipsychotic medications also provide some evidence for the benefit of medication.

Box 10.1 summarizes some of the rationale for psychotropic medication.

Box 10.1 Rationale for use of psychotropic medication

- High prevalence of psychiatric disorders in people who die by suicide
- A low proportion of people who die by suicide have been prescribed medication
- Some RCT evidence of reduction of suicidal ideation with antidepressants
- Pharmaco-epidemiological evidence of the effectiveness of SSRI antidepressants, the mood stabilizer lithium, and the antipsychotic clozapine in reducing suicide.

10.3 Antidepressants

10.3.1 Randomized controlled trial evidence

Because of the relatively low base rate of suicide, it is not feasible to conduct RCTs to demonstrate a reduction in suicide as a standalone outcome. However, some RCTs of antidepressants versus placebo have demonstrated statistically significant reductions in suicidal ideation (Szanto et al., 2003). Meta-analytic studies of antidepressants versus placebo have shown a weak association between selective serotonin reuptake inhibitor (SSRI) antidepressant use and an increased risk of non-fatal self-harm, but not suicide (Fergusson et al., 2005; Gunnell et al., 2005). This association may not be specific to SSRI antidepressants, with similar effects being found with tricyclic antidepressants (Jick et al., 2004).

It is interesting that emerging suicidality similar to that reported in drug trials has also been described in non-pharmacological psychotherapy treatment of depressed adolescents (Bridge et al., 2005). In one comparison between medication and psychotherapy, SSRI antidepressants were actually associated with a *lower* risk of treatment-emergent suicidal ideation than interpersonal psychotherapy (Rucci et al., 2011). It is also worth noting that reports of unexpected suicide deaths during the early period of recovery from depression have been reported for almost two hundred years (Goldney, 2007)—a time period which of course predates drug treatment.

In studies which have shown increased suicidal behaviour associated with medication use, part of the explanation may be 'confounding by indication'—there is a degree of suicide risk associated with all psychiatric disorders and those most likely to receive medication may be those at highest risk.

10.3.2 Pharmaco-epidemiological studies

A pioneering programme to enhance the recognition and treatment of depression by general practitioners on the Swedish island of Gotland was followed by a decrease in suicide, a greater use of antidepressants, a decreased prescription of antipsychotics and hypnotics, a decrease in inpatient treatment of depression, and a reduction in sick leave due to depression (Rutz et al., 1992). Further important work has emerged from Sweden, where a naturalistic experiment was made possible by the fact that antidepressant prescribing increased threefold. This change was associated with a reduction in suicide. Similar associations were found in the other Nordic countries, and this was hailed as a 'medical breakthrough' in suicide prevention (Isacsson, 2000).

However, the findings from ecological studies internationally have been more mixed (Baldessarini et al., 2007). In one review, only nine of 29 ecological studies reported significant correlations between increased use of antidepressants and declining suicide rates. There is less evidence for the effectiveness of antidepressants in children and adolescents than there is for adults. Nevertheless, pharmaco-epidemiological data of their suicide prevention potential has been reported from the USA, where a significant negative correlation between antidepressant treatment and suicide in different regions was found. It was calculated that a 1 per cent increase in adolescent use of antidepressants was associated with a decrease of 0.23 suicide deaths per 100,000 adolescents each year (Olfson et al., 2003). Also relevant is the effect of regulatory warnings about antidepressant use. Gibbons et al. found that reductions in antidepressant use in adolescents after the warnings were issued were associated with increases in suicide (Gibbons et al., 2007).

These findings suggesting that the treatment of depression has an impact on suicide are not unexpected in view of the clinical risk factors described previously.

However, it has only been by large population studies, rather than by RCTs, that the impact on suicide has been demonstrated. Apart from a power issue (RCTs are generally too small to look at suicide as an outcome), this might also reflect the fact that people with suicidal thoughts or behaviours are commonly excluded from antidepressant treatment trials.

The generally positive observational data has not convinced all who have been concerned about reports of suicidal behaviour being precipitated by SSRI antidepressants, particularly in the young. Of course, the potential risks of treatment compared to its benefits need to be considered. The overall number needed to harm for adults is about one in 700 (Fergusson et al., 2005) and about one in 120 for children and adolescents (Brent, 2009). In terms of benefit, the number needed to treat for significant improvement is between one in four to one in seven for adults (Gunnell et al, 2005), and one in 10 for children and adolescents (Brent, 2009). What this suggests is that more than a hundred times as many adults would benefit from antidepressants than would experience suicidal thoughts and behaviours; and that 12 times as many children and adolescents would do so. The potential benefit of careful antidepressant use in some young people is accepted by clinicians and generally endorsed by clinical guidelines (Maalouf and Brent, 2012).

A review of large observational studies of post-mortem toxicology in young people who had died by suicide may further allay concerns about the extent to which SSRI use is associated with suicide (Dudley et al., 2010). Six studies from the UK, Denmark, Sweden, and the USA examined the use of SSRIs in association with suicide in young persons. In combining the data from these studies (and considering the prevalence of depression in association with suicide in the young) it was striking that only nine (1.6 per cent) out of 574 young people who died by suicide had evidence of SSRI use in association with their death. Such a finding is inconsistent with the hypothesis that SSRI antidepressants are likely to precipitate suicide, but it is consistent with other studies that have demonstrated inadequate recognition and treatment of depression in those who die by suicide, no matter what their age.

When antidepressants are used, it is imperative that an adequate dose be prescribed. It is also essential to be aware not only of the possible risk of suicide, but of the potential risk of not treating those who are depressed and suicidal. A collaborative approach to prescribing, and close monitoring and supervision are essential. Less toxic antidepressants should be prescribed because of the risk of overdose. It is also important that the duration of treatment is adequate. The general consensus is that antidepressants should be used for at least six months in patients with a first episode of depression, and prescribers should consult the latest clinical guidelines (e.g. National Institute of Health and Care Excellence (NICE) or British Association of Psychopharmacology (BAP) guidelines in the UK, Royal Australian and New Zealand College of Psychiatrists (RANZCP) guidelines in Australia, American Psychiatric Association (APA) guidelines in the USA) for advice on maintenance treatment. Some observational studies have suggested that antidepressants may be less effective in depressed patients who have suicidal thoughts than those who do not (Lopez-Castroman et al., 2016), and so other treatments (e.g. psychological interventions—see Chapter 9) should be considered in conjunction.

10.4 Ketamine

Ketamine is a short-acting anaesthetic and sometimes used as a recreational drug. It is a NMDA receptor antagonist. When administered in low doses it appears to have very rapid but short-term antidepressant and antisuicidal effects. One recent randomized trial (N = 80) compared intravenous infusions of ketamine versus midazolam in depressed patients with suicidal ideation. Over half of patients (55 per cent) showed a clinically important improvement in suicidal ideas in the ketamine group compared to less than one third (30 per cent) in the midazolam group (Grunebaum et al., 2018). The effects were maintained for six weeks. Most investigations have involved intravenous administration, but a nasal delivery route has also been developed and a number of randomized trials are underway. Of course, further studies testing risks and benefits are necessary, but ketamaine may have promise for the treatment of suicidal thoughts and behaviours particularly in the emergency department setting (Lee et al., 2015). Ketamine has also recently been granted a restricted licence for treatment-resistant depression in the USA.

10.5 Lithium and other mood stabilizers

A number of studies have reported a reduction in suicide with use of lithium in patients with affective disorders. One review reported that early naturalistic observations of 1.5, 1.3, and 0.7 suicide deaths per thousand patient years in three studies of persons on long-term lithium treatment were markedly lower than the estimated 5.1 to 11.6 suicide deaths per thousand patient years in untreated unipolar and bipolar illnesses (Goldney, 2005). Other reviews have added weight to those reports.

A meta-analysis of 31 studies (involving 85,229 person years of follow-up) concluded that the overall risk of suicide and attempted suicide was five times less among lithium-treated patients than those not treated with lithium (Baldessarini et al., 2006). Another meta-analysis of 48 RCTs found that lithium treatment was associated with reduced risk of suicide and other causes of death (ORs (95%CI): 0.13 (0.03 to 0.66) and 0.38 (0.15 to 0.95) respectively). There was a protective effect in people with unipolar depression as well as bipolar affective disorder (Cipriani et al., 2013).

It has also been estimated that although lithium probably prevents about 250 suicide deaths per year in Germany, only 0.06 per cent of the German population were prescribed lithium. If one assumes both a conservative estimate of the prevalence of bipolar disorders and also that only half would be prescribed lithium, then rational treatment would dictate that prescription rates of lithium should be approximately 10 times higher (Muller-Oerlinghausen et al., 2005). Similarly, a UK study showed that at least 40 per cent of patients with bipolar disorder who died by suicide were not prescribed lithium or a mood stabilizer (Clements et al., 2013).

Other anticonvulsants and mood stabilizers may not have the same suicide prevention properties. In a retrospective cohort study of 20,638 health-plan members with bipolar disorder (Goodwin et al., 2003), suicide and suicide attempts were 2.7 and 1.7 times higher, respectively, with sodium valproate compared to lithium treatment. A review of other studies found no protective effect for valproate, carbamazepine, or lamotrigine (Oquendo et al., 2005).

Overall, the best available evidence is that the mood stabilizer of choice to tackle suicidality is lithium. Naturally this choice needs to be considered in the context of the tolerability of side effects, adherence issues, monitoring, and patient acceptability. Intriguingly there is some evidence that the very low doses of naturally occurring lithium in drinking water may also be associated with reduced suicide incidence (Vita et al., 2015)

10.6 Antipsychotic medication

Observations in the mid-1990s in the USA suggested that antipsychotic-resistant patients treated with clozapine for between six months and seven years (mean 3.5 years) had 'markedly less suicidality' than non-clozapine-treated patients (Meltzer et al., 2003). Attempted suicide decreased from 25 per cent to 3.5 per cent; the lethality of suicide attempts which did occur was reduced; suicidal intent was reduced; and there was a significant decrease in hopelessness. There were similar findings from another American study of 30,000 patients with schizophrenia and schizoaffective disorder, with clozapine-treated patients having a suicide rate of 12.7 per 100,000 per year compared to 63.1 per 100,000 per year for all patients with those disorders in the USA (Reid et al., 1998).

These findings led to an ambitious multi-centre trial in 67 centres in 11 countries, comparing clozapine with the atypical antipsychotic olanzapine (Meltzer et al., 2003). A total of 980 patients with schizophrenia or schizoaffective disorder were randomized to the treatments, and non-pharmacological input was identical. Clozapine was significantly more effective in reducing suicide attempts, hospitalization, and the need for emergency intervention, but the suicide deaths were too few for statistical analysis. It was evident that clozapine was more effective than olanzapine, regardless of any individual risk factor such as substance abuse or number of previous suicide attempts. Since then a meta-analysis has reported that long-term treatment with clozapine is associated with a threefold reduction in suicidal behaviour and suicide (Hennen and Baldessarini, 2005).

As clozapine is usually reserved for those with resistance to conventional antipsychotic medication, these studies are persuasive. However, it cannot be assumed that the so-called atypical antipsychotics as a whole are more effective in reducing suicidality than older medications, particularly with the Clinical Antipsychotic Trials of Intervention Effectiveness (CATIE) study demonstrating few differences in outcome between the 'newer' (atypical) and older preparations (Owens, 2008). Nevertheless, there is now more reason to believe that vigorous treatment of schizophrenia, particularly with clozapine, has the potential to reduce the likelihood of suicidal behaviours. Of course treatment with clozapine necessitates regular haematological monitoring because of the risk of blood dyscrasias.

10.7 Adherence

Medication can be prescribed by the clinician but it must also be taken by the patient. Data from the UK National Confidential Inquiry into Suicide and Homicide suggests that 13 per cent of patients who died by suicide were not taking medication as prescribed in the month before death (National Confidential Inquiry into Suicide and Homicide by People with Mental Illness, 2017). If adherence to medication is an issue, steps should be taken to understand reasons why this is the case, and intervention arranged as appropriate. Effective approaches may include talking through the rationale for medication, psychoeducation, specific psychological interventions, and medication reviews (Ehret and Wang, 2013). Family involvement may also be helpful. If these measures fail, compulsory treatment orders (as appropriate to the local jurisdiction) might sometimes be necessary. By the time such approaches are being considered, community mental health workers are likely to be involved. However, it is still important for each patient to have a family practitioner who co-ordinates overall management, particularly when community mental health services now predominate in many countries. The family practitioner has traditionally been in a good position to provide continuity of care. However, primary care is under pressure itself in many settings.

10.8 Conclusion

It should be reiterated that medications are not prescribed specifically to prevent suicide, but to treat the psychiatric disorders associated with suicidal behaviour. They are simply one component of the standard care which should be provided by a modern health service. Good communication, collaborative prescribing, patient choice, and close supervision are important general principles. Figure 10.1 is an infographic summarizing the information in this chapter.

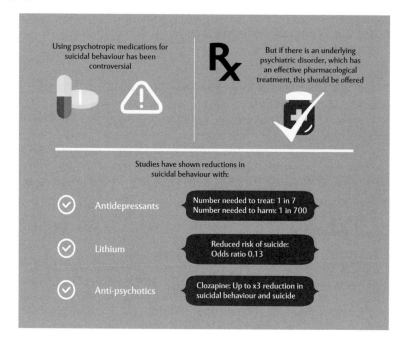

Fig 10.1 **Pharmacological approaches to suicide prevention.**
Courtesy of Dr Sarah Steeg.

REFERENCES

Angst, F., Stassen, H. H., Clayton, P. J., and Angst, J. (2002). Mortality of patients with mood disorders: follow-up over 34–38 years. *J Affect Disord* **68**(2–3): 167–81.

Baldessarini, R. J., Tondo, L., Davis, P., Pompili, M., Goodwin, F. K., and Hennen, J. (2006). Decreased risk of suicides and attempts during long-term lithium treatment: a meta-analytic review. *Bipolar Disord* **8**(5 Pt 2): 625–39.

Baldessarini, R. J., Tondo, L., Strombom, I. M., et al. (2007). Ecological studies of antidepressant treatment and suicidal risks. *Harv Rev Psychiatry* **15**(4): 133–45.

Barraclough, B. (1972). Suicide prevention, recurrent affective disorder and lithium. *Br J Psychiatry* **121**(563): 391–2.

Brent, D. A. (2009). Selective serotonin reuptake inhibitors and suicidality: a guide for the perplexed. *Can J Psychiatry* **54**(2): 72–4; discussion 75.

Bridge, J. A., Barbe, R. P., Birmaher, B., Kolko, D. J., and Brent, D. A. (2005). Emergent suicidality in a clinical psychotherapy trial for adolescent depression. *Am J Psychiatry* **162**(11): 2173–5.

Cipriani, A., Hawton, K., Stockton, S., and Geddes, J. R. (2013). Lithium in the prevention of suicide in mood disorders: updated systematic review and meta-analysis. *BMJ* **346**: f3646.

Clements, C., Morriss, R., Jones, S., Peters, S., Roberts, C., and Kapur, N. (2013). Suicide in bipolar disorder in a national English sample, 1996–2009: frequency, trends and characteristics. *Psychol Med* **43**(12): 2593–602.

Dudley, M., Goldney, R., and Hadzi-Pavlovic, D. (2010). Are adolescents dying by suicide taking SSRI antidepressants? A review of observational studies. *Australas Psychiatry* **18**(3): 242–5.

Ehret, M. J. and Wang, M. (2013). How to increase medication adherence: what works? *Ment Health Clin* **2**(8): 230–2.

Fergusson, D., Doucette, S., Glass, K. C., et al. (2005). Association between suicide attempts and selective serotonin reuptake inhibitors: systematic review of randomised controlled trials. *BMJ* **330**(7488): 396.

Gibbons, R. D., Brown, C. H., Hur, K., et al. (2007). Early evidence on the effects of regulators' suicidality warnings on SSRI prescriptions and suicide in children and adolescents. *Am J Psychiatry* **164**(9): 1356–63.

Goldney, R. D. (2005). Suicide prevention: a pragmatic review of recent studies. *Crisis* **26**(3): 128–40.

Goldney, R. D. (2007). An historical note on suicide during the course of treatment for depression. *Suicide Life Threat Behav* **37**(1): 116–17.

Goodwin, F. K., Fireman, B., Simon, G. E., Hunkeler, E. M., Lee, J., and Revicki, D. (2003). Suicide risk in bipolar disorder during treatment with lithium and divalproex. *JAMA* **290**(11): 1467–73.

Grunebaum, M. F., Galfalvy, H. C., Choo, T. H., et al. (2018). Ketamine for rapid reduction of suicidal thoughts in major depression: a midazolam-controlled randomized clinical trial. *Am J Psychiatry* **175**(4): 327–35.

Gunnell, D., Saperia, J., and Ashby, D. (2005). Selective serotonin reuptake inhibitors (SSRIs) and suicide in adults: meta-analysis of drug company data from placebo controlled, randomised controlled trials submitted to the MHRA's safety review. *BMJ* **330**(7488): 385.

Hennen, J. and Baldessarini, R. J. (2005). Suicidal risk during treatment with clozapine: a meta-analysis. *Schizophr Res* **73**(2–3): 139–45.

Isacsson, G. (2000). Suicide prevention—a medical breakthrough? *Acta Psychiatr Scand* **102**(2): 113–17.

Jick, H., Kaye, J. A., and Jick, S. S. (2004). Antidepressants and the risk of suicidal behaviors. *JAMA* **292**(3): 338–43.

Lee, J., Narang, P., Enja, M., and Lippmann, S. (2015). Use of ketamine in acute cases of suicidality. *Innov Clin Neurosci* **12**(1–2): 29–31.

Lopez-Castroman, J., Jaussent, I., Gorwood, P., and Courtet, P. (2016). Suicidal depressed patients respond less well to antidepressants in the short term. *Depress Anxiety* **33**(6): 483–94.

Maalouf, F. T. and Brent, D. A. (2012). Child and adolescent depression intervention overview: what works, for whom and how well? *Child Adolesc Psychiatr Clin N Am* 21(2): 299–312, viii.

Marzuk, P. M., Tardiff, K., Leon, A. C., et al. (1995). Use of prescription psychotropic drugs among suicide victims in New York City. *Am J Psychiatry* 152(10): 1520–2.

Meltzer, H. Y., Alphs, L., Green, A. I., et al. (2003). Clozapine treatment for suicidality in schizophrenia: International Suicide Prevention Trial (InterSePT). *Arch Gen Psychiatry* 60(1): 82–91.

Muller-Oerlinghausen, B., Felber, W., Berghofer, A., Lauterbach, E., and Ahrens, B. (2005). The impact of lithium long-term medication on suicidal behavior and mortality of bipolar patients. *Arch Suicide Res* 9(3): 307–19.

National Confidential Inquiry into Suicide and Homicide by People with Mental Illness (2017). *Annual report: England, Northern Ireland, Scotland and Wales*. From http:// documents.manchester.ac.uk/display.aspx?DocID=37560

Olfson, M., Shaffer, D., Marcus, S. C., and Greenberg, T. (2003). Relationship between antidepressant medication treatment and suicide in adolescents. *Arch Gen Psychiatry* 60(10): 978–82.

Oquendo, M. A., Chaudhury, S. R., and Mann, J. J. (2005). Pharmacotherapy of suicidal behavior in bipolar disorder. *Arch Suicide Res* 9(3): 237–50.

Owens, D. C. (2008). What CATIE did. Some thoughts on implications deep and wide'. *Psychiatr Serv* 59: 530–3.

Reid, W. H., Mason, M., and Hogan, T. (1998). Suicide prevention effects associated with clozapine therapy in schizophrenia and schizoaffective disorder. *Psychiatr Serv* 49(8): 1029–33.

Rucci, P., Frank, E., Scocco, P., et al. (2011). Treatment-emergent suicidal ideation during 4 months of acute management of unipolar major depression with SSRI pharmacotherapy or interpersonal psychotherapy in a randomized clinical trial. *Depress Anxiety* 28(4): 303–9.

Rutz, W., von Knorring, L., and Walinder, J. (1992). Long-term effects of an educational program for general practitioners given by the Swedish Committee for the Prevention and Treatment of Depression. *Acta Psychiatr Scand* 85(1): 83–8.

Szanto, K., Mulsant, B. H., Houck, P., Dew, M. A., and Reynolds III, C. F. (2003). Occurrence and course of suicidality during short-term treatment of late-life depression. *Arch Gen Psychiatry* 60(6): 610–17.

Vita, A., De Peri, L., Sacchetti, E. Lithium in drinking water and suicide prevention: a review of the evidence. *Int Clin Psychopharmacol* 2015; 30: 1–5.

The role of health services and systems

KEY POINTS

- Many individuals have been in contact with health services prior to suicide. Specialist mental health services are important, but primary care, general hospitals, and community settings have a role too.
- Service-wide changes (e.g. crisis care, dual-diagnosis services, serious incident reviews) can contribute to suicide prevention.
- Focusing on safety in particular settings (e.g. inpatient care) can also be highly effective.
- Clinical guidelines can improve the quality of care and outcomes for patients, but implementation is key.
- Safer systems of care (with a number of interventions introduced simultaneously) may reduce suicide.

11.1 Clinical and systems-based approaches to suicide prevention

Suicide and suicidal behaviour may sometimes be conceptualized as societal problems with a wide range of underlying contributory factors. Only a minority of individuals are in contact with mental health professionals before death, so it could be argued that specialist services only have a limited role to play in preventing suicide. However, we know that many who die by suicide may have an underlying mental disorder. Those people in contact with services are a very important group who in many cases are seeking help for their distress. Clinical approaches are also helpful because a focus on suicide prevention in mental health services generally leads to safer care for all. Of course, clinical approaches involve more than just specialist mental health services: for example, primary care or the general hospital. Taking this wider perspective, many people have been in contact with some form of health service prior to suicide. In this chapter, we will focus on the contribution of health services to suicide prevention as well as discuss the role of systems-based approaches to prevention, where several interventions are implemented simultaneously.

11.2 Safety in mental health services

In the late twentieth century, a number of countries introduced broad suicide-prevention strategies, which will be referred to in Chapter 12. Even prior to releasing a formal strategy in the UK, a more focused initiative—the National

> **Box 11.1** National policies and safety recommendations from the National Confidential Inquiry into Suicide and Homicide (2001)
>
> • Removal of ligature points from inpatient settings
> • Provision of assertive outreach teams
> • 24-hour crisis teams available
> • Follow up within seven days of discharge from psychiatric inpatient care
> • Responding to non-compliance
> • Policies for dual-diagnosis patients
> • Information sharing with criminal justice systems
> • Multidisciplinary reviews after adverse incidents
> • Training in the assessment and management of suicide risk.

Confidential Inquiry into Suicide by People with Mental Illness—was introduced. This involved collecting detailed information from clinical teams on all people who died by suicide within 12 months of specialist mental health contact. It has been running for more than 20 years and there are currently 30,000 patients on the database. The data have been used to improve health services and systems of care.

11.2.1 The role of national policies and recommendations

As a result of early work, the National Confidential Inquiry made a series of wide ranging recommendations designed to improve patient safety (see Box 11.1) (National Confidential Inquiry into Suicide and Homicide by People with Mental Illness, 2001). There were two important questions from a national policy perspective. The first was whether these service changes were implemented? The second (and more important question) was whether these changes made any difference to patient care and ultimately suicide rates?

With respect to the first question, when all mental health services in England and Wales were surveyed, self-report data certainly seemed to indicate that the changes were being implemented. As to whether the changes were making a difference to suicide rates, services that implemented more of the recommendations seemed to be safer in terms of lower suicide incidence. Suicide rates before and after implementation of each of the nine service changes were also examined. For three of the service changes in particular there were big falls in suicide: implementation of 24-hour crisis care; having a dual-diagnosis policy (a marker of clinical activity in this area); and having a system of multidisciplinary review after suicide (perhaps an indicator of a learning culture). These falls were not observed in services which did not implement the changes. The reduction in suicide was clinically important—these service changes were associated with 200–300 fewer suicide deaths per year (While et al., 2012)

11.2.2 Focusing on safety in particular settings

In common with some other countries, inpatient beds in the UK have reduced in number and the focus of care has moved to the community, with crisis-resolution home treatment (CRHT) being provided. This is an alternative intensive community-based service for managing high-risk patients in their homes. The National Confidential Inquiry data allowed a comparison of suicide rates in crisis teams and inpatient care. There was a reduction in suicide rates for both treatment settings, but the rate was consistently lower for inpatient treatment than for CRHT, as illustrated in Figure 11.1.

It was reassuring that there was a decrease in suicide in both settings, and it could not be accounted for simply by falling general population suicide rates or changes in case mix. There have been large reductions in deaths by hanging on the ward and patients who die after absconding, suggesting at least some positive impact of the safety recommendations. However, the lower rate for inpatient care was perhaps surprising, as the now smaller inpatient population might be expected to have higher levels of morbidity. The corollary is that with more acutely unwell persons having CRHT in the community, there would be an increased number of suicide deaths in that setting (which in fact was the case), but the actual suicide rate (taking into account the larger number of patients receiving CRHT) went down.

This differential suicide rate between the two settings is of some concern, although the analysis did not take into account time at risk. The study suggests that criteria for community treatment should be explored and perhaps revised. At the very least it emphasizes the need to monitor all parts of the system to ensure

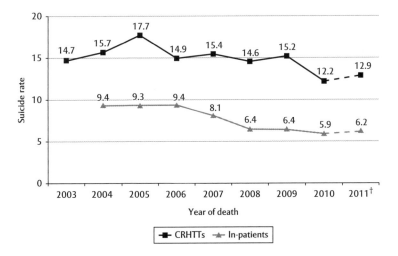

Fig 11.1 Rate of suicide among community patients under crisis-resolution home treatment (per 10,000 episodes) and inpatients (per 10,000 admissions), England 2003*–2011.

* MHMDS data were not complete in 2003; therefore, inpatient suicide rates are presented for 2004–2011 only.
† Data completeness for patient suicides by year was 81–99 per cent. Figures in 2011 have been uplifted by a factor so that the estimated numbers reflect the average completeness of all years (97 per cent).
Adapted from *Lancet Psychiatry*, 1, Hunt IM, Rahman MS, While D, et al. Safety of patients under the care of crisis resolution home treatment services in England: a retrospective analysis of suicide trends from 2003 to 2011, pp. 135–141. Copyright © 2014 Elsevier Ltd. All rights reserved. doi:https://doi.org/10.1016/S2215-0366(14)70250-0.

that the problem of high suicide rates in one service (e.g. inpatient care) does not simply shift elsewhere (e.g. crisis teams).

11.2.3 Organizational context

Organizational context is of major importance when it comes to patient safety. An examination of which organizational factors were associated with suicide in mental health services found no important association with factors such as staff and patient satisfaction, staff sickness, or patient complaints (Kapur et al., 2016). However, non-medical staff turnover (turnover of nursing staff and other allied health professionals) did appear to be associated with suicide rates: suicide was more frequent in those mental health services with a greater staff turnover. Why might staff turnover be associated with poor safety? Of course this could be a chance association. It could also be that a high staff turnover is a marker of a failing organization which is badly run as well as having safety issues and concerns. But the relationship might also be causal in that staff who are not in post for very long will not get to know patients well. They will be unable to provide the same continuity of care as a stable workforce, and this could compromise safety.

Interestingly, implementing service changes in services which are organization-ally healthy seems to have much more of an impact than implementing them in services with organizational problems (Kapur et al., 2016). In other words, changes to mental health services will really only have the desired impact if they are made in well-run organizations. We need to attend to both individual service factors and the organizational context in which care is provided in order to improve patient safety. Rather than thinking solely of *individual service changes* or *individual inter-ventions* it is more helpful to also implement better and *safer systems of care*. The work of the National Confidential Inquiry over two decades suggests a number of measures that might be taken together in order to improve safety in mental health services (The National Confidential Inquiry into Suicide and Homicide by People with Mental Illness, 2016) (see Figure 11.2 at the end of this chapter).

11.3 Primary care and the wider context

Health-service contact before suicide is not restricted to psychiatric services. Data from the UK show that in the year prior to suicide, around a quarter of people have been seen by mental health services (The National Confidential Inquiry into Suicide and Homicide by People with Mental Illness, 2017), nearly 40 per cent have been seen in emergency departments (Gairin et al., 2003). and 60–70 per cent have been seen by their general practitioners (Windfuhr et al., 2016). About one third have had no clinical contact. Therefore, considering suicide prevention in a wider health-service and community context is likely to be helpful.

11.3.1 Multi-component interventions

While it is fair to say that most of the early national programmes (which will be discussed in Chapter 12) embodied a broad approach to suicide prevention, there have been a number of more focused multi-component interventions.

A study of the introduction of a community-based programme in a cohort of over five million USA air-force personnel (Knox et al., 2003) had some striking findings. The study focused on reducing the stigma associated with seeking help for psychosocial problems, enhancing mental health literacy, and changing administrative policies to facilitate access to intervention services. There was a 33 per cent reduction in suicide between the time periods 1990 to 1996 and 1997 to 2002. There was also a decrease in accidental death, homicide, and family violence, which is not unexpected as they share many of the antecedents of suicidal behaviours.

Positive results were also reported from Germany in the Nuremberg Alliance Against Depression study, where a two-year campaign to inform people about depression, train family doctors, and encourage co-operation with community facilitators (e.g. teachers, priests, the media, self-help groups) resulted in a statistically significant reduction in suicidal behaviour in Nuremberg compared with a control region in Wuerzburg (which did not participate in the programme) (Hegerl et al., 2006). There were some concerns about the comparability of intervention and control regions, but the results were promising. Encouraging results were also reported from other regions of Germany and Hungary. An enhanced intervention, the Optimising Suicide Prevention Programs and Their Implementation in Europe (OSPI Europe)—combining elements of the Alliance Against Depression work with other strategies—has been tested in Ireland, Portugal, Germany, and Hungary and has been reported to show some benefit (Hegerl et al., 2009, 2013).

A study from Canada of a comprehensive suicide prevention programme with the Montreal police force reported a 79 per cent reduction in suicide compared with a rise of 11 per cent in other police regions in Quebec which did not have the programme (Mishara and Martin, 2012). The programme involved education of all units, their supervisors, and their union representatives, the provision of a confidential designated telephone helpline, and a publicity campaign with articles in internal police magazines as well as posters and brochures in police units.

A Japanese study examined a community-based multimodal intervention consisting of local government leadership, public awareness and education, and gatekeeper training, designed to support high-risk groups. The study reported potential benefits, with a reduction in suicidal behaviour in rural areas and in men (Ono et al., 2013).

A comprehensive, multimodal American programme, focused on suicide prevention in young people aged 16–23 years, included gatekeeper training, education and mental health awareness, screening, improved community partnership working, interventions for people bereaved by suicide, and crisis hotlines (Garraza et al., 2015). The intervention was tested in over 460 intervention sites and compared to usual practice in over 1,100 control sites. The researchers found that in the first year the intervention areas had significantly lower rates of attempted suicide than the control areas (4.9 fewer attempts per 1,000 youths). However, although the programme continued, they acknowledged that there was no evidence of longer-term differences in suicide attempt rates.

A recent report of a cluster randomized trial of a multilevel intervention in New Zealand failed to find an impact on suicide rates (Collings et al., 2018). The intervention consisted of training in recognition of suicide risk factors, workshops on mental health, community-based intervention, and distribution of information. The authors suggested that the lack of impact might have been due to the context (well-developed existing services, and a national context that was different from earlier studies), the fact that the intervention was not focused on depression, inadequate power, poor implementation, or contamination between intervention and control regions. It was also possible, they speculated, that the promise of multimodal interventions might have been overstated.

The aforementioned studies from several different countries demonstrate the diverse manner in which multi-component suicide-prevention approaches can be implemented in a broader context. All are evidence-based, in the sense that their individual components have been subjected to some scrutiny. However, the overall outcomes have been variable. Two other recently instituted programmes, with slightly different approaches, are being followed with interest.

Zero Suicide was developed in the USA and is based on a system of 'perfect depression care' which focuses on healthcare organizations. It includes restriction of access to means of suicide, screening and assessment for mental disorders, systematic care protocols, and enhanced support during transition between services. The labelling of this approach as 'Zero Suicide' has been questioned but endorsed by Mokkenstorm et al., who emphasized organizational commitment as a key element (Mokkenstorm et al., 2018). Ambitious targets may have a galvanizing effect, but they also have the potential to deepen feelings of failure and guilt in family, friends, clinicians, and services when suicide deaths do occur. Indeed, even the best clinical care within a supportive administrative system cannot guarantee that all suicide deaths will be prevented. A large-scale evaluation of the model is currently being undertaken in several centres in the USA (Ahmedani, 2017).

An Australian intervention, LifeSpan, comprises a number of components co-ordinated and delivered through primary healthcare networks at the community level. These include improving the identification of people in distress and their pathways to care, reducing access to means of suicide, working with the media, and improving the competency and confidence of frontline workers in dealing with people in a suicidal crisis. A wider community approach to prevention is integral (Baker et al., 2018). Proponents suggest that successful implementation may achieve a 20 per cent reduction in suicide deaths and 30 per cent reduction in attempted suicide.

It is important to emphasize that evaluations of multi-component interventions are complex, methodologically challenging, expensive, and may be difficult to interpret. It is not often clear what the 'active ingredient' of a helpful intervention might be. Collings et al. argue that future studies must be carefully designed and clearly reported, including contextual information about local health systems and pre-existing prevention activities (Collings et al., 2018).

11.3.2 The role of primary care

The role of primary care in suicide prevention is under-researched. In a large study carried out in UK general practice (Windfuhr et al., 2016), researchers found that the average general practice experienced one suicide death every two years and that suicide was an uncommon occurrence for individual general practitioners (GPs). The study also found that 60–70 per cent of people who died by suicide had seen their GP in the year before death. This might have represented an opportunity to intervene. People who did not consult at all were at increased risk of suicide compared to those who consulted once, but those who consulted frequently were at particularly high risk of suicide. There were low rates of medication prescription and specialist referral prior to suicide. Other studies have found that rates of self-harm recorded in primary care are high and strongly associated with premature mortality (Carr et al., 2017).

A primary-care study focusing on better recognition and treatment of depression in older patients showed promising results (Almeida et al., 2012). This cluster randomized controlled trial involved 373 primary-care physicians and 21,762 patients aged 60 years or older. The intervention was a practice audit with personalized feedback, printed educational material, and six-monthly educational newsletters over a period of two years (compared to a practice audit and newsletters alone). The researchers found that the intervention reduced the prevalence of depressive symptoms and self-harm by 10 per cent at two years in patients treated by physicians in the intervention group compared to those treated by control-group physicians. Other primary care based approaches could address the suicide risk associated with physical conditions and alcohol-related problems (McDowell et al., 2011; Webb et al., 2012).

Health-service strategies can be utilized in those who attend healthcare facilities, but the groups who do not attend (e.g. middle-aged men) present a particular challenge. Strategies for this group could include increasing awareness of and access to mental healthcare perhaps by providing information and services at sporting events or community settings, or through voluntary rather than statutory mental health services (National Confidential Inquiry into Suicide and Homicide by People with Mental Illness, 2014).

11.4 The role of clinical guidelines

What part might clinical guidelines play in the prevention of suicide? In England, the National Institute for Health and Care Excellence (NICE) issues guidance for all clinicians. In 2004, they published guidance on the short-term management of people who harmed themselves. A national study sought to examine whether the guidelines had had an effect on management by comparing the interventions and treatment people received in 32 hospitals in England in 2001–2002 to that received in 2010–2011 (Cooper et al., 2013). The results were disappointing. The rates of mental health assessment remained similar, the rates of mental health aftercare actually went down, and rates of psychiatric admission and primary-care referral stayed very much the same. The rates of medical admission did in fact go up, but this was really a 'policy artefact'—around this time a target was introduced into the health service which suggested that no patient should wait longer than four hours in an emergency department, as a result of which many patients were admitted to short-stay wards. Despite these rather disappointing findings, there was some evidence that the quality of care, as measured by a global quality score, may have improved between the two time periods.

In 2012, NICE published updated guidance on the longer-term management of self-harm (National Collaborating Centre for Mental Health, 2012). Although this represents detailed high-quality evidence-based guidance, implementation always remains a challenge. Partly to address this implementation gap, NICE have also introduced a system of measurable quality standards which identify components of high-quality care. These are outlined in Box 11.2. NICE has recently published guidelines on suicide prevention in both community and custodial settings (National Institute for Health and Care Excellence, 2018).

Improving the implementation of guidance is an important goal. A recent nationwide cluster RCT from the Netherlands recruited 45 psychiatry departments and 880 patients (de Beurs et al., 2015). The intervention consisted of structured face-to-face training sessions delivered to whole clinical teams, with e-learning to improve guideline adherence. The study examined the effect both on clinicians and the patients treated by those clinicians. As might be expected, the investigators found better guideline adherence, as well as improved knowledge and confidence,

---

Box 11.2 NICE quality statements for self-harm services

Statement 1. People who have self-harmed are cared for with compassion and the same respect and dignity as any service user.

Statement 2. People who have self-harmed have an initial assessment of physical health, mental state, safeguarding concerns, social circumstances and risks of repetition or suicide.

Statement 3. People who have self-harmed receive a comprehensive psychosocial assessment.

Statement 4. People who have self-harmed receive the monitoring they need while in the healthcare setting, in order to reduce the risk of further self-harm.

Statement 5. People who have self-harmed are cared for in a safe physical environment while in the healthcare setting, in order to reduce the risk of further self-harm.

Statement 6. People receiving continuing support for self-harm have a collaboratively developed risk management plan.

Statement 7. People receiving continuing support for self-harm have a discussion with their lead healthcare professional about the potential benefits of psychological interventions specifically structured for people who self-harm.

Statement 8. People receiving continuing support for self-harm and moving between mental health services have a collaboratively developed plan describing how support will be provided during the transition.

amongst the clinicians who had had the training compared to those who had not. Although they did not find an impact on overall suicidal ideation or future attempts in the patients themselves, they did find a possible effect in the subgroup of patients with depression. This is a novel and important study because it shows that training clinicians can potentially impact on the care their patients receive and ultimately their outcomes. This trial needs replicating in other settings.

11.5 Conclusion

Healthcare providers have an important part to play in suicide prevention. Patients being treated by mental health services may be at particularly high risk of suicide, but primary care and acute medical services also have a role. Implementing several interventions simultaneously and thinking in terms of safer 'systems' of care, rather than at the level of the individual patient or an individual treatment, might be a powerful approach. Such strategies need further testing in research studies. At the very least, it is important that both the individual and systems approaches embody the highest standards of evidence-based care (Large and Kapur, 2018). Figure 11.2 is an infographic summarizing the information in this chapter.

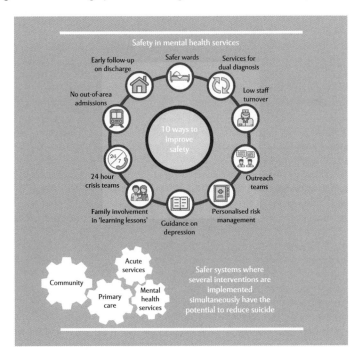

Fig 11.2 The role of health services and systems in suicide prevention.
Courtesy of Dr Sarah Steeg.

REFERENCES

Ahmedani, B. (2017). *An Evaluation of the Zero Suicide Model Across Learning Healthcare Systems*. From http://hcsrn.org/mhrn/en/ResearchProjects/ZeroSuicide.html

Almeida, O. P., Pirkis, J., Kerse, N., et al. (2012). A randomized trial to reduce the prevalence of depression and self-harm behavior in older primary care patients. *Ann Fam Med* **10**(4): 347–56.

Baker, S. T., Nicholas, J., Shand, F., Green, R., and Christensen, H. (2018). A comparison of multi-component systems approaches to suicide prevention. *Australas Psychiatry* **26**(2): 128–31.

Carr, M. J., Ashcroft, D. M., Kontopantelis, E., et al. (2017). Premature death among primary care patients with a history of self-harm. *Ann Fam Med* **15**(3): 246–54.

Collings, S., Jenkin, G., Stanley, J., McKenzie, S., and Hatcher, S. (2018). Preventing suicidal behaviours with a multilevel intervention: a cluster randomised controlled trial. *BMC Public Health* **18**(1): 140.

Cooper, J., Steeg, S., Bennewith, O., et al. (2013). Are hospital services for self-harm getting better? An observational study examining management, service provision and temporal trends in England. *BMJ Open* **3**(11): e003444.

de Beurs, D. P., Bosmans, J. E., de Groot, M. H., et al. (2015). Training mental health professionals in suicide practice guideline adherence: cost-effectiveness analysis alongside a randomized controlled trial. *J Affect Disord* **186**: 203–10.

Gairin, I., House, A., and Owens, D. (2003). Attendance at the accident and emergency department in the year before suicide: retrospective study. *Br J Psychiatry* **183**: 28–33.

Garraza, L. G., Walrath, C., Goldston, D. B., Reid, H., and McKeon, R. (2015). Effect of the Garrett Lee Smith Memorial Suicide Prevention Program on suicide attempts among youths. *JAMA Psychiatry* **72**(11): 1143–9.

Hegerl, U., Althaus, D., Schmidtke, A., and Niklewski, G. (2006). The alliance against depression: 2-year evaluation of a community-based intervention to reduce suicidality. *Psychol Med* **36**(9): 1225–33.

Hegerl, U., Rummel-Kluge, C., Varnik, A., Arensman, E., and Koburger, N. (2013). Alliances against depression—a community based approach to target depression and to prevent suicidal behaviour. *Neurosci Biobehav Rev* **37**(10 Pt 1): 2404–9.

Hegerl, U., Wittenburg, L., Arensman, E., et al. (2009). Optimizing Suicide Prevention Programs and Their Implementation in Europe (OSPI Europe): an evidence-based multi-level approach. *BMC Public Health* **9**(1): 428.

Hunt, I. M., Rahman, M. S., While, D., et al. (2014). Safety of patients under the care of crisis resolution home treatment services in England: a retrospective analysis of suicide trends from 2003 to 2011. *Lancet Psychiatry* **1**(2): 135–41.

Kapur, N., Ibrahim, S., While, D., et al. (2016). Mental health service changes, organisational factors, and patient suicide in England in 1997–2012: a before-and-after study. *Lancet Psychiatry* **3**(6): 526–34.

Knox, K. L., Litts, D. A., Talcott, G. W., Feig, J. C., and Caine, E. D. (2003). Risk of suicide and related adverse outcomes after exposure to a suicide prevention programme in the US Air Force: cohort study. *BMJ* **327**(7428): 1376.

CHAPTER 11

Large, M. M. and Kapur, N. (2018). Psychiatric hospitalisation and the risk of suicide. *Br J Psychiatry* **212**(5): 269–73.

McDowell, A. K., Lineberry, T. W., and Bostwick, J. M. (2011). Practical suicide-risk management for the busy primary care physician. *Mayo Clin Proc* **86**(8): 792–800.

Mishara, B. L. and Martin, N. (2012). Effects of a comprehensive police suicide prevention program. *Crisis* **33**(3): 162–8.

Mokkenstorm, J. K., Kerkhof, A., Smit, J. H., and Beekman, A. T. F. (2018). Is it rational to pursue zero suicides among patients in health care?' *Suicide Life Threat Behav* **48**(6): 745–54.

National Collaborating Centre for Mental Health (2012). Self-Harm: Longer-Term Management. Leicester: British Psychological Society.

National Confidential Inquiry into Suicide and Homicide by People with Mental Illness(2001). *Safety First:Five-Year Report of the National Confidential Inquiry into Suicide and Homicide by People with Mental Illness.* London: Department of Health Publications.

National Confidential Inquiry into Suicide and Homicide by People with Mental Illness (2014). *Suicide in Primary Care in England: 2002–2011.* From http://documents. manchester.ac.uk/display.aspx?DocID=37574

National Confidential Inquiry into Suicide and Homicide by People with Mental Illness(2016). *Making Mental Health Care Safer.* From http://documents.manchester. ac.uk/display.aspx?DocID=37580

National Confidential Inquiry into Suicide and Homicide by People with Mental Illness (2017). *Annual Report: England, Northern Ireland, Scotland and Wales.* From http:// documents.manchester.ac.uk/display.aspx?DocID=37560

National Institute for Health and Care Excellence (2018). *Preventing Suicide in Community and Custodial Settings.* From https://www.nice.org.uk/guidance/ng105

Ono, Y., Sakai, A., Otsuka, K., et al. (2013). Effectiveness of a multimodal community intervention program to prevent suicide and suicide attempts: a quasi-experimental study. *PLoS One* **8**(10): e74902.

Webb, R. T., Kontopantelis, E., Doran, T., Qin, P., Creed, F., and Kapur, N. (2012). Suicide risk in primary care patients with major physical diseases: a case-control study. *Arch Gen Psychiatry* **69**(3): 256–64.

While, D., Bickley, H., Roscoe, A., et al. (2012). Implementation of mental health service recommendations in England and Wales and suicide rates, 1997–2006: a cross-sectional and before-and-after observational study. *Lancet* **379**(9820): 1005–12.

Windfuhr, K., While, D., Kapur, N., et al. (2016). Suicide risk linked with clinical consultation frequency, psychiatric diagnoses and psychotropic medication prescribing in a national study of primary-care patients. *Psychol Med* **46**(16): 3407–17.

Preventing suicide through population-based approaches

> **KEY POINTS**
>
> - Restriction of access to means of suicide is effective but usually requires legislation to introduce at a national level.
> - Responsible media reporting can help to prevent some suicide deaths.
> - Other population-based strategies, for example those designed to reduce the availability of alcohol, reduce the stigma of help-seeking, increase public spending, may also be effective.
> - National programmes of suicide prevention are needed to have a major impact on suicide.

12.1 Individual versus population-based approaches

Individual interventions by individual clinicians undoubtedly have the potential to save lives, but many of the biggest health gains have been made by public health measures applied across whole populations. This is potentially an extremely powerful strategy (Rose, 1992). In this chapter we will discuss some of the most important population-based approaches for suicide prevention.

12.2 Restriction of access to means of suicide

Restriction of access to means is probably the most effective suicide-prevention measure of all. Why might this be? Although death by suicide is often the result of multiple and complex causes, the final act may be impulsive. One of the hall-marks of suicidal behaviour is ambivalence—uncertainty about the wish to live or die. Preventing access to a potentially lethal means of suicide can buy time during which suicidal ideas may subside and become less intense. Substitution with other lethal means can occur but probably only does so in a minority of in-dividuals. There are a number of examples illustrating that restriction of access to the means of suicide is a highly effective suicide-prevention measure and these are listed in Box 12.1.

12.2.1 Historical context

The 'coal gas story' in the UK refers to the detoxification of domestic gas sup-plies (natural North Sea gas with a lower carbon monoxide content replaced

---

Box 12.1 Effective restriction of access to means of suicide

- Barbiturate-prescribing legislation
- The 'coal gas story', catalytic convertors, and restricting access to barbeque charcoal
- Barriers to jumping—bridges, car parks
- Restrictingavailability of pesticides
- Analgesic legislation
- Firearms restriction.

---

gas manufactured from coal) which resulted in a sustained reduction in suicide of about 30 per cent (Kreitman, 1976). This was associated with a modest increase in suicide by other means, such as poisoning (Gunnell et al., 2000), particularly in the younger age groups, but that increase was relatively small, and much smaller than the overall reduction in suicide. This is powerful evidence to refute the argument that there is no point in restricting access to the means of suicide as a person with suicidal intent will simply switch to an alternative method.

12.2.2 High-frequency locations

Being in close proximity to railways, bridges, and other similar sites is associated with suicide risk. Sometimes sites become well known and even attract those who are suicidal. Restricting access is effective. There was a clear demonstration of this principle in a study from New Zealand, where a natural experiment of removing and reinstalling safety barriers—in essence an A–B–A research design—showed that the barriers were effective in preventing suicide: their removal increased suicide; and their reinstatement prevented suicide (Beautrais et al., 2009). Barriers on the Clifton Suspension Bridge in England were associated with a halving of the suicide rate, with no displacement to nearby sites (Bennewith et al., 2007). There are numerous other examples from the world literature. Apart from restricting access, other strategies that might be effective at high-frequency locations include encouraging help-seeking (e.g. providing helpline numbers) and increasing the likelihood of intervention from others (e.g. CCTV cameras) (Pirkis et al., 2015).

12.2.3 Medication

One of the first examples of the effect of reducing medication availability was the report of a reduction in suicide due to barbiturate poisoning in Australia following the blister packaging of medication and restriction on the number of tablets/capsules that could be prescribed (Oliver and Hetzel, 1972). In England and Wales, a common method of suicide has been the ingestion of paracetamol (acetaminophen). This was targeted by legislation to restrict pack sizes available to buy 'over the counter'. There was a 43 per cent reduction in suicide deaths (representing 765 fewer deaths) in the 11 years following the legislation (Hawton et al., 2012). There was also a 60 per cent reduction in registrations for liver transplantation due to paracetamol-induced hepatotoxicity. Another example is the substantial reduction in suicide mortality (500 fewer deaths over five years) following regulatory withdrawal of an opiate analgesic, coproxamol, with little indication of substitution with other painkillers (Hawton et al., 2012).

12.2.4 Pesticides

In low- and middle-income countries, the ready availability of highly lethal pesticides is being addressed. A recent study from Sri Lanka showed that the phased bans of pesticides were associated with a 50 per cent reduction in pesticide suicide and a 21 per cent reduction in the overall rate of suicide between 2011 and 2015 (Knipe et al., 2017). A review of the worldwide literature suggests that bans are probably more effective than sales restrictions (Gunnell et al., 2017), and a groundbreaking randomized trial of over 50,000 households and 200,000 individuals suggested that restricting access by storing pesticides in locked boxes was not an effective strategy to prevent deaths (Pearson et al., 2017). It should also be noted that, to date, this is the largest randomized trial in the whole field of suicide prevention.

12.2.5 Firearms

Firearms are the most common cause of suicide in the USA, and although there is unequivocal case-control evidence of an association between the possession of firearms in a household and an increased risk of suicide, wider cultural attitudes (e.g. the belief in the right to bear arms) is a stumbling block to legislative change. However, in those regions where there has been restrictive legislation, there has been an associated reduction in suicide, and this has also been demonstrated in a number of other countries including Canada, Australia, New Zealand, and Austria (Lewiecki and Miller, 2013). Furthermore, a case-control study has demonstrated that storing a firearm in a locked location, storing it unloaded, ensuring the ammunition is locked, and storing the ammunition separately, are each associated with a protective effect (Grossman et al., 2005).

12.2.6 Carbon monoxide

Carbon monoxide poisoning by motor vehicle exhaust fumes has been a common method of suicide in some countries and is potentially preventable (Ostrom et al., 1996). Catalytic converters—an environmental measure rather than a suicide-prevention measure—have minimized the risk. In England, legislation requiring all new cars to be fitted with catalytic convertors in 1993 was associated with a halving in the proportion of suicide deaths by car exhaust asphyxiation (Amos et al., 2001). An Australian study found that areas with a higher concentration of older vehicles had higher rates of suicide by motor vehicle exhaust gas (Studdert et al., 2010).

Carbon monoxide poisoning by burning barbeque charcoal in a sealed room has become a common method of suicide in some Far Eastern countries. Chang and colleagues showed a marked increase in incidence in suicide from this method from 1995 to 2011 in Hong Kong, Taiwan, Japan, the Republic of Korea, and Singapore (Chang et al., 2014). Restricting access by removing bags of charcoal from open sale to locked storage, and community action (to identify people with suspicious buying habits, or refusing holiday rentals to distressed individuals), may be associated with fewer deaths (Yip et al., 2012).

12.2.7 Hanging

Hanging is the most common form of suicide in a number of countries including the UK and Australia. The means are widely available and not subject to potential legislation or restriction outside of institutional settings. Since around 20 per cent of hanging deaths occur in controlled environments, such as prisons or hospitals, the potential overall impact of intervention is limited. Nevertheless, ligature points should be eliminated in custodial and treatment settings (Gunnell et al., 2005).

One very important and perhaps neglected issue is cognitive availability—why do people chose this method? Why is it an option for them? A qualitative study found that it was perceived as relatively painless (Biddle et al., 2010). It is possible that population-based and individual initiatives could be utilized to influence this perception (Mok et al., 2012). These could include avoiding media portrayal of this method as quick and painless, and also clinicians sensitively asking about choice of methods with people who are suicidal. This is an extremely difficult area and of course the danger is that, for some people, it increases knowledge and awareness of the method and inadvertently promotes cognitive availability.

12.2.8 Means restriction: problems and practicalities

The restriction of access to means of suicide is probably effective not only because of the preclusion of a lethal method per se, but also because it buys time. The final suicidal impulse may dissipate. Substitution, however, does occur in some (probably a minority) of individuals (Daigle, 2005). Substitution may be less common in women, older people, and in low- and middle-income countries. It is also important to emphasize that most of these public-health initiatives to reduce access to means of suicide require legislation and the political will to introduce them. They might be considered intrusive by some members of the community. Yip and colleagues (2012) suggest some criteria for policy makers to consider before implementing means restriction (Yip et al., 2012). The focus should be on common high-lethality methods (otherwise there is a danger that people may substitute methods that are even more lethal); the methods should be amenable to restriction; the strategy may be more effective if the method is high-profile and socially recognized; and it should be feasible to monitor the method accurately.

It is probably fair to say that national approaches related to minimizing access to the means of suicide have the potential for the greatest influence on suicide rates worldwide. One challenge, of course, is to remain vigilant for newer methods of suicide as they appear (e.g. novel forms of gassing) and to take appropriate action (Gunnell et al., 2015).

12.3 Media reporting of suicide

The 'Werther effect' refers to the increase in suicide after the publication of a novel by Goethe in the eighteenth century in which a young man (Werther) died by suicide. Since then it has generally been accepted that publicity about suicide results in further such deaths. However, probably the first study to convincingly demonstrate a possible causal association between the media and suicide was a German analysis of suicide following the presentation of a TV series that depicted the death, by railway suicide, of a 19-year-old man (Schmidtke and Hafner, 1988). Against advice this was repeated, thereby allowing a naturalistic A–B–A–B–A research design. Following both screenings there was an increase in imitative suicide, with the greatest and most enduring increase being in those persons closest in age to the main character.

Since then, other research has demonstrated unequivocally that there is an association between publicity about suicide and subsequent increases in suicidal behaviour. A study in the USA found that suicide deaths in young people that attracted more newspaper reports were more likely to be followed by a cluster of suicide deaths than suicides in young people which attracted less reporting (Gould et al., 2014). A recent statistical investigation focusing on the reporting of a possible cluster of suicide deaths in young people in Wales concluded there was indeed a cluster, but it was smaller and later than that reported in the media. In fact, the cluster began after early media reports, which raises the possibility that the media portrayal may have been responsible for propagating it (Jones et al., 2013).

Poor reporting is associated with an increase in suicidal behaviour, but the media may also have a role in preventing suicide by promoting mental-health initiatives. There is the additional dilemma of balancing freedom of the press with social responsibility. Guidelines for responsible reporting about suicide have been developed in conjunction with media organizations and professionals (Sisask and Varnik, 2012; Samaritans, 2013; WHO, 2017). These guidelines also consider the welfare and needs of friends and family bereaved by the suicide deaths. Common elements are listed in Box 12.2.

Co-operation with the media does have an effect on reporting and this was demonstrated by an analysis of newspapers in Switzerland after guidelines had been drawn up. The proportion of suicide deaths featuring on newspaper front pages reduced from 20 per cent to 4 per cent. For stories which did report on

Box 12.2 Guidelines for media reporting of suicidal behaviour

- Avoiding detailed description of the means of suicide
- Not sensationalizing reporting, idealizing the deceased, or giving stories undue prominence (e.g. no large headlines or front-page news)
- Avoiding stigmatizing terms (e.g. 'suicide epidemic', 'hotspot', 'commit suicide'—suicide has been decriminalized for many years in most Western countries)
- Including details of support groups and sources of help
- Avoiding any reference to pro-suicide sites or websites which provide detail on particular methods of suicide
- Reporting that suicide is usually associated with a remediable mental health problem, recognizing the complexities of suicide, and avoiding reference to final triggering events
- Considering the effect on bereaved relatives.

deaths, the proportion including sensational headlines reduced from 62 per cent to 25 per cent (Michel et al. 2000).

One of the first examples of effective suicide prevention by restriction of media reporting was in Vienna, where responsible reporting of suicide deaths on the subway resulted in an 80 per cent reduction in the number of such deaths (Etzersdorfer and Sonneck, 1998). Other studies from Austria have also reported the favourable impact of media guidelines, with there being a significant reduction in suicide in regions where collaborating newspapers had a large population coverage (Etzersdorfer et al., 2004; Niederkrotenthaler and Sonneck, 2007).

Responsible reporting can minimize the adverse effect of media publicity, but can the media also make a positive contribution to the prevention of suicide in its own right? Volunteer organizations such as the Samaritans and other crisis centres rely on media publicity, as do some mental-health education programmes. Mass media awareness-raising campaigns can be helpful. They may be most useful when delivered as part of a suite of interventions, but the messaging of such campaigns requires careful consideration (Pirkis et al., 2017). The 'Papageno effect' is named after a character in Mozart's opera 'The Magic Flute' whose suicidal crisis was averted by the intervention of other characters. In an interesting analysis of the type of media reports which might increase suicidal behaviour (the Werther Effect) as opposed to decrease it (the Papageno effect), researchers suggested that stories which depicted people in crisis using coping strategies other than suicidal behaviour were associated with lower suicide rates (Niederkrotenthaler et al., 2010).

12.3.1 Responding to suicide clusters

The strict definition of a cluster varies depending on the context in which it occurs. With regard to suicide, it refers to the occurrence of more suicide deaths than expected (usually three or more) during a particular time period or in a particular location, or both. Some authors make a distinction between 'point clusters', where there may be a direct connection between people concerned, and 'mass clusters', where the suicide deaths may be exposed to a common factor such as widespread media reporting (Joiner, 1999). Of course some clusters will be a mixture of the two.

The media may play a particular role in the aftermath of a cluster, since one major concern is imitative behaviour or contagion. Responding to a cluster is challenging. One approach is to develop a community action plan with a multi-disciplinary team to facilitate the accurate provision of information, the careful management of media reporting, and access to help for people who need it most (Public Health England, 2015).

12.3.2 The internet, social media, and suicide

The role of internet and social media with respect to suicidal behavior is receiving increasing attention, much of it negative (Luxton et al., 2012). Examples include the provision of detailed information on methods of suicide (Biddle et al., 2008), cyberbullying leading to suicide, suicide pacts, and websites and social media communities which normalize or even encourage suicidal behaviour while discouraging help-seeking.

But there are positive aspects as well. Many websites promote suicide prevention. A recent systematic review highlighted how social media can reach large numbers of people who might otherwise be very hard to engage. Potentially it also offers a means to intervene. Sites may provide a supportive and helpful space in which people can discuss suicidal thoughts and behaviours without fear of being judged. Challenges include ensuring that user behaviour is moderated, managing risk, confidentiality, and avoiding contagion (Robinson et al., 2016).

More research is clearly needed on the positive and negative aspects of social media use, including who might benefit most and who might be most vulnerable. Legislation and regulation may be part of the answer, but controlling access or content across borders is challenging. Such strategies may also conflict with the principle of freedom of expression, lack of censorship, and the idea of the web as an unregulated creative space. User education is of course important and there is an increasing emphasis on online safety, particularly in young people.

12.3.3 Suicide prevention and e-health

There has been much interest in the potential role of suicide-prevention computer programs, tools, or apps for smartphones and other digital devices. Although one systematic review concluded that the evidence base was weak and the effects were of uncertain clinical significance, it did suggest that digital interventions might be associated with a reduction in suicidal ideation (Witt et al., 2017). An overview of the content of available apps found that just under half included an interactive suicide-prevention feature such as obtaining support from family and friends, making a safety plan to act upon, measures to restrict access to means, and facilitating access to crisis services (Larsen et al., 2016). The authors concluded that no apps provided comprehensive evidence-based support and some included potentially harmful content (such as details of methods of suicide or encouraging risk-taking during times of crisis).

An innovative series of trials involving around four hundred participants recruited via the web, tested an app against an active control (Franklin et al., 2016). The intervention—therapeutic evaluative conditioning (TEC)— was a game-like app which involved pairing stimuli in order to increase aversion to self-injurious thoughts and behaviours and decrease aversion to self. The intervention was associated with reductions in self-reported cutting, suicide plans, and suicidal behaviours during the month for which participants had access to the app. However, there was no effect on suicide ideation and no persistence of the treatment effect at one-month follow-up.

This is an extremely active and rapidly developing research area which will yield important findings and new tools in the coming years. Online or mobile-phone-based safety planning (see Chapter 9) is another active area of research.

12.4 School-based approaches to suicide prevention

A systematic review examined school-based prevention programmes. There was a general lack of high-quality evidence but interventions such as 'Signs of Suicide' (a suicide awareness and education programme) and the 'good behaviour game' (a classroom-based behavioural management approach to improve self-regulation) appear to reduce suicide attempts (Katz et al., 2013). Forms of gatekeeper training (where professionals such as teachers are taught to recognize the signs and symptoms of suicidal behaviour) may also have promise. However, a recent major multinational school-based randomized trial suggested that a programme of youth awareness and peer support reduced suicide attempts compared to the non-intervention control group, but gatekeeper training or screening by professionals may have been less effective (Wasserman et al., 2015).

12.5 Other population-based approaches

Potentially there are other population-based strategies to prevent suicide which may target underlying risk factors rather than suicidal behaviours themselves. For example, reductions in alcohol consumption following pricing, legislative, or social change may be associated with lower suicide rates (Pridemore et al., 2013). Economic and social policies may also have a role. In a landmark paper, Stuckler and colleagues suggested that countries which increased rather than decreased welfare spending at a time of global recession protected themselves against an increase in suicide seen elsewhere (Stuckler et al., 2009). The authors argued that 'recessions hurt but austerity kills'. Population-based strategies which aim to reduce the stigma of mental illness and promote help-seeking may also have a role to play in the prevention of suicide (Rusch et al., 2014).

12.6 National policies and programmes

Governments were comparatively slow to appreciate the enormous impact of suicidal behaviour, not only at the individual level but at the population level as well. The first national approach was in 1985, when Finnish health authorities introduced a programme aiming to lower the suicide rate by 20 per cent over the following ten years (Kerkhof, 1999). In fact, suicide increased initially, but then reduced to a figure about 9 per cent below the baseline figure. The programme was research-based and involved community education about risk factors, with guidelines for health promotion provided for schools, the armed forces, and clergy, as well as the social care sector. In an evaluation, it was acknowledged that there had been a division between the medical model and sociocultural paradigms in understanding and preventing suicidal behaviour. It was suggested that more attention could have been paid to reducing access to means of suicide and to suicide prevention in the elderly (Kerkhof, 1999). Nevertheless, it was considered that the project did contribute to the reduction in suicide rate.

A number of other countries have since introduced national programmes. These tend to have certain common elements which have been summarized in a World Health Organization framework for a public health approach to suicide prevention (WHO, 2012). By 2014, WHO estimated that 28 countries had national strategies, and the number was growing (WHO, 2014).

One example is the suicide prevention strategy for England, originally launched in 2002 and updated in 2012 (Department of Health, 2012). The strategy includes six areas for action (see Box 12.3). There were further updates in 2016, with a strengthened focus on men, self-harm, and support for bereaved families

---

Box 12.3 Areas for action of the Suicide Prevention Strategy for England

- Reduce suicide in key high-risk groups
- Improve mental health in specific population groups
- Reduce access to the means of suicide
- Better information and support for those bereaved by suicide
- Support the media in delivering sensitive approaches to reporting
- Support research, data collection, and monitoring.

(Department of Health, 2017). The areas for action include most aspects of suicide prevention and are informed by much of the research discussed in this and previous chapters. It is reassuring that there were substantial reductions in suicide in England between 2002 and 2008 (the onset of the recession), and also more recently.

Falls associated with the implementation of suicide prevention strategies have also been reported in other countries: for example, in the USA and Australia rates reduced by almost 30 per cent from their peak in 1997 to 2004, and there was a reduction of about 50 per cent in suicide in young men aged 15–24 years (Goldney, 2006). Debate arose about what may have been the effective components, and one study concluded that improved detection and management of depression may have played a role (Hall et al., 2003). However, the complexity of determining the exact reason for that reduction in suicide is demonstrated by the sobering observation that the change in young men was confined to the middle and higher socioeconomic groups, and the historical predominance of suicide deaths in rural areas actually increased (Page et al., 2007). Clearly, the broad programme in Australia did not reach everyone in the community, even though the overall impact was positive. More recently there have been concerns about rising rates of suicide in some groups.

National interventions could be criticized for their over-general nature and the lack of specific theoretical frameworks. Zalsman and colleagues reviewed recent international research examining the effectiveness of suicide prevention strategies (Zalsman et al., 2016). They considered 23 systematic reviews, 12 meta-analyses, 40 randomized trails, 67 cohort studies, and 22 ecological studies. They found good evidence for the effectiveness of reducing the availability of lethal methods of suicide (e.g. analgesics, restricting access to high-frequency locations), and some evidence for school-based and pharmacological approaches (e.g. antidepressants, clozapine, lithium) and psychological approaches (e.g. CBT). The effects of screening in primary care, awareness raising, and media guidelines were uncertain. The authors highlighted the overall lack of RCTs in this field and suggested that gatekeeper training, physician education, helplines, and internet-based interventions needed further research.

12.7 Conclusion

Population-based interventions such as restricting access to lethal means of suicide and improving media reporting are powerful suicide prevention strategies. They may be challenging to implement and evaluate. RCTs are often not feasible. However, as helpful as population-based approaches are, they are not a panacea. The careful assessment and management of the individual suicidal person remains important. National strategies which draw these individual and public health components together are needed to have a major impact on suicide. Figure 12.1 is an infographic summarizing the information in this chapter.

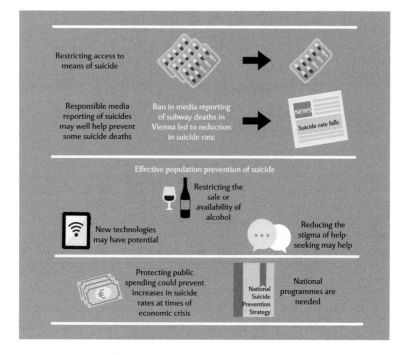

Fig 12.1 Population-based approaches to suicide prevention.
Courtesy of Dr Sarah Steeg.

REFERENCES

Amos, T., Appleby, L., and Kiernan, K. (2001). Changes in rates of suicide by car exhaust asphyxiation in England and Wales. *Psychol Med* **31**(5): 935–9.

Beautrais, A. L., Gibb, S. J., Fergusson, D. M., Horwood, L. J., and Larkin, G. L. (2009). Removing bridge barriers stimulates suicides: an unfortunate natural experiment. *Aust N Z J Psychiatry* **43**(6): 495–7.

Bennewith, O., Nowers, M., and Gunnell, D. (2007). Effect of barriers on the Clifton Suspension Bridge, England, on local patterns of suicide: implications for prevention. *Br J Psychiatry* **190**: 266–7.

Biddle, L., Donovan, J., Hawton, K., Kapur, N., and Gunnell, D. (2008). Suicide and the internet. *BMJ* **336**(7648): 800–2.

Biddle, L., Donovan, J., Owen-Smith, A., et al. (2010). Factors influencing the decision to use hanging as a method of suicide: qualitative study. *Br J Psychiatry* **197**(4): 320–5.

Chang, S. S., Chen, Y. Y., Yip, P. S., Lee, W. J., Hagihara, A., and Gunnell, D. (2014). Regional changes in charcoal-burning suicide rates in East/Southeast Asia from 1995 to 2011: a time trend analysis. *PLoS Med* **11**(4): e1001622.

Daigle, M. S. (2005). Suicide prevention through means restriction: assessing the risk of substitution. A critical review and synthesis. *Accid Anal Prev* **37**(4): 625–32.

Department of Health (2012). Preventing Suicide in England. A Cross-Government Outcomes Strategy to Save Lives. From https://assets.publishing.service.gov. uk/government/uploads/system/uploads/attachment_data/file/430720/ Preventing-Suicide-.pdf

Department of Health (2017). *Preventing Suicide in England: Third Progress Report of the Cross-Government Outcomes Strategy to Save Lives.* From https://assets.publishing. service.gov.uk/government/uploads/system/uploads/attachment_data/file/582117/ Suicide_report_2016_A.pdf

Etzersdorfer, E. and Sonneck, G. (1998). Preventing suicide by influencing mass-media reporting. The Viennese experience 1980–1996. *Arch Suicide Res* **4**(1): 67–74.

Etzersdorfer, E., Voracek, M., and Sonneck, G. (2004). A dose–response relationship between imitational suicides and newspaper distribution. *Arch Suicide Res* **8**(2): 137–45.

Franklin, J. C., Fox, K. R., Franklin, C. R., et al. (2016). A brief mobile app reduces nonsuicidal and suicidal self-injury: evidence from three randomized controlled trials. *J Consult Clin Psychol* **84**(6): 544–57.

Goldney, R. (2006). Suicide in Australia: some good news. *Med J Aust* **185**: 304.

Gould, M. S., Kleinman, M. H., Lake, A. M., Forman, J., and Midle, J. B. (2014). Newspaper coverage of suicide and initiation of suicide clusters in teenagers in the USA, 1988–96: a retrospective, population-based, case-control study. *Lancet Psychiatry* **1**(1): 34–43.

Grossman, D. C., Mueller, B. A., Riedy, C., et al. (2005). Gun storage practices and risk of youth suicide and unintentional firearm injuries. *JAMA* **293**(6): 707–14.

Gunnell, D., Bennewith, O., Hawton, K., Simkin, S., and Kapur, N. (2005). The epidemiology and prevention of suicide by hanging: a systematic review. *Int J Epidemiol* **34**(2): 433–42.

Gunnell, D., Coope, C., Fearn, V., et al. (2015). Suicide by gases in England and Wales 2001–2011: evidence of the emergence of new methods of suicide. *J Affect Disord* **170**: 190–5.

Gunnell, D., Knipe, D., Chang, S. S., et al. (2017). Prevention of suicide with regulations aimed at restricting access to highly hazardous pesticides: a systematic review of the international evidence. *Lancet Glob Health* **5**(10): e1026–e1037.

Gunnell, D., Middleton, N., and Frankel, S. (2000). Method availability and the prevention of suicide—a re-analysis of secular trends in England and Wales 1950–1975. *Soc Psychiatry Psychiatr Epidemiol* **35**(10): 437–43.

Hall, W. D., Mant, A., Mitchell, P. B., Rendle, V. A., Hickie, I. B., and McManus, P. (2003). Association between antidepressant prescribing and suicide in Australia, 1991–2000: trend analysis. *BMJ* **326**(7397): 1008.

Hawton, K., Bergen, H., Simkin, S., Wells, C., Kapur, N., and Gunnell, D. (2012). Six-year follow-up of impact of co-proxamol withdrawal in England and Wales on prescribing and deaths: time-series study. *PLoS Med* **9**(5): e1001213.

Joiner, T. E. (1999). The clustering and contagion of suicide. *Curr Dir Psychol Sci* **8**(3): 89–92.

Jones, P., Gunnell, D., Platt, S., et al. (2013). Identifying probable suicide clusters in Wales using national mortality data. *PLoS One* **8**(8): e71713.

Katz, C., Bolton, S. L., Katz, L. Y., et al. (2013). A systematic review of school-based suicide prevention programs. *Depress Anxiety* **30**(10): 1030–45.

Kerkhof, A. J. (1999). The Finnish national suicide prevention program evaluated. *Crisis* **20**(2): 50–63.

Knipe, D. W., Chang, S. S., Dawson, A., et al. (2017). Suicide prevention through means restriction: impact of the 2008–2011 pesticide restrictions on suicide in Sri Lanka. *PLoS One* **12**(3): e0172893.

Kreitman, N. (1976). The coal gas story. United Kingdom suicide rates, 1960–71. *Br J Prev Soc Med* **30**(2): 86–93.

Larsen, M. E., Nicholas, J., and Christensen, H. (2016). A systematic assessment of smartphone tools for suicide prevention. *PLoS One* **11**(4): e0152285.

Lewiecki, E. M. and Miller, S. A. (2013). Suicide, guns, and public policy. *Am J Public Health* **103**(1): 27–31.

Luxton, D. D., June, J. D., and Fairall, J. M. (2012). Social media and suicide: a public health perspective. *Am J Public Health* **102**(**Suppl 2**): S195–200.

Michel, K., Frey, C., Wyss, K., and Valach, L. (2000). An exercise in improving suicide reporting in print media. *Crisis* **21**(2): 71–9.

Mok, P. L., Kapur, N., Windfuhr, K., et al. (2012). Trends in national suicide rates for Scotland and for England & Wales, 1960–2008. *Br J Psychiatry* **200**(3): 245–51.

Niederkrotenthaler, T. and Sonneck, G. (2007). Assessing the impact of media guidelines for reporting on suicides in Austria: interrupted time series analysis. *Aust N Z J Psychiatry* **41**(5): 419–28.

Niederkrotenthaler, T., Voracek, M., Herberth, A., et al. (2010). Role of media reports in completed and prevented suicide: Werther v. Papageno effects. *Br J Psychiatry* **197**(3): 234–43.

Oliver, R. G. and Hetzel, B. S. (1972). Rise and fall of suicide rates in Australia: relation to sedative availability. *Med J Aust* **2**(17): 919–23.

Ostrom, M., Thorson, J., and Eriksson, A. (1996). Carbon monoxide suicide from car exhausts. *Soc Sci Med* **42**(3): 447–51.

Page, A., Morrell, S., Taylor, R., Dudley, M., and Carter, G. (2007). Further increases in rural suicide in young Australian adults: secular trends, 1979–2003. *Soc Sci Med* **65**(3): 442–53.

Pearson, M., Metcalfe, C., Jayamanne, S., et al. (2017). Effectiveness of household lockable pesticide storage to reduce pesticide self-poisoning in rural Asia: a community-based, cluster-randomised controlled trial. *Lancet* **390**(10105): 1863–72.

Pirkis, J., Rossetto, A., Nicholas, A., Ftanou, M., Robinson, J., and Reavley, N. (2017). Suicide prevention media campaigns: a systematic literature review. *Health Commun*: 1–13.

Pirkis, J., Too, L. S., Spittal, M. J., Krysinska, K., Robinson, J., and Cheung, Y. T. (2015). Interventions to reduce suicides at suicide hotspots: a systematic review and meta-analysis. *Lancet Psychiatry* **2**(11): 994–1001.

Pridemore, W. A., Chamlin, M. B., and Andreev, E. (2013). Reduction in male suicide mortality following the 2006 Russian alcohol policy: an interrupted time series analysis. *Am J Public Health* **103**(11): 2021–6.

Public Health England (2015). *Identifying and Responding to Suicide Clusters and Contagion. A Practice Resource*. London: Department of Health.

Robinson, J., Cox, G., Bailey, E., et al. (2016). Social media and suicide prevention: a systematic review. *Early Interv Psychiatry* **10**(2): 103–21.

Rose, G. (1992). *Rose's Strategy of Preventive Medicine*. Oxford: Oxford University Press.

Rusch, N., Zlati, A. Black, G., and Thornicroft, G. (2014). Does the stigma of mental illness contribute to suicidality? *Br J Psychiatry* **205**(4): 257–9.

Samaritans. (2013). *Media Guidelines for Reporting Suicide*. From https://www.samaritans.org/media-centre/media-guidelines-reporting-suicide

Schmidtke, A. and Hafner, H. (1988). The Werther effect after television films: new evidence for an old hypothesis. *Psychol Med* **18**(3): 665–76.

Sisask, M. and Varnik, A. (2012). Media roles in suicide prevention: a systematic review. *Int J Environ Res Public Health* **9**(1): 123–38.

Stuckler, D., Basu, S., Suhrcke, M., Coutts, A., and McKee, M. (2009). The public health effect of economic crises and alternative policy responses in Europe: an empirical analysis. *Lancet* **374**(9686): 315–23.

Studdert, D. M., Gurrin, L. C., Jatkar, U., and Pirkis, J. (2010). Relationship between vehicle emissions laws and incidence of suicide by motor vehicle exhaust gas in Australia, 2001–06: an ecological analysis. *PLoS Med* **7**(1): e1000210.

Wasserman, D., Hoven, C. W. Wasserman, C., et al. (2015). School-based suicide prevention programmes: the SEYLE cluster-randomised, controlled trial. *Lancet* **385**(9977): 1536–44.

Witt, K., Spittal, M. J., Carter, G., et al. (2017). Effectiveness of online and mobile telephone applications ('apps') for the self-management of suicidal ideation and self-harm: a systematic review and meta-analysis. *BMC Psychiatry* **17**(1): 297.

World Health Organization (2012). *Public Health Action for the Prevention of Suicide: A Framework*. From http://apps.who.int/iris/bitstream/handle/10665/75166/?sequence=1

World Health Organization (2014). *Preventing Suicide: A Global Imperative 2014*. From http://www.who.int/mental_health/suicide-prevention/world_report_2014/en/

World Health Organization (2017). *Preventing Suicide: A Resource for Media Professionals—Update 2017*. From http://www.who.int/mental_health/suicide-prevention/resource_booklet_2017/en/

Yip, P. S., Caine, E., Yousuf, S., Chang, S. S., Wu, K. C., and Chen, Y. Y. (2012). Means restriction for suicide prevention. *Lancet* **379**(9834): 2393–9.

Zalsman, G., Hawton, K., Wasserman, D., et al. (2016). Suicide prevention strategies revisited: 10-year systematic review. *Lancet Psychiatry* **3**(7): 646–59.

CHAPTER 13

Bereavement after suicide

KEY POINTS

- Supporting people bereaved by suicide should be a key component of suicide prevention strategies.
- People bereaved by suicide may be at increased risk of suicidal behaviour but are less likely to obtain support than other bereaved groups.
- There may be qualitative differences in the issues or grief themes which arise when someone is bereaved through suicide compared to those which arise after death from other causes.
- Clinicians are vulnerable to similar feelings as well as being subject to concerns about their professional competence.
- Information resources, psychological interventions, and support groups may be helpful for people bereaved by suicide.

13.1 Introduction

After someone dies by suicide, multiple people suffer intense grief. Although the number was underestimated in the past (Grad, 2011), contemporary work suggests that around 60 people may be affected by each suicide death (Pitman et al., 2014). This means that every year there are probably at least 50 million people worldwide who are affected by suicide. However, a recent American study suggested that the number of people touched by a suicide death might be as high as 135 (Cerel et al., 2019), which means the global figure would be in excess of one million. The importance of bereavement by suicide has been recognized internationally by its inclusion in many suicide prevention policies. In England, for example, it is now one of the major themes in the new strategy.

Traditionally, suicide has been regarded as being commonly associated with complicated grief in those left behind, but recent work suggests that grief reactions vary greatly. We should also note that much of the research in this area is from high-income settings. There is a need for studies of bereavement in low- and middle-income countries.

13.2 Quantitative studies

Suicide bereavement has been a focus of a number of recent epidemiological studies and findings suggest that people who are bereaved by suicide are themselves at higher risk. A Danish population-based study of people aged 25–60 years who had died by suicide found that spousal bereavement was associated with a high risk of suicide, especially for men, who had a nearly fiftyfold increase in risk compared to the general population (Agerbo, 2005). Loss of a child through suicide was also associated with an elevated risk. A later study compared people bereaved following the death of their spouse by suicide with people whose spouse had died from other causes (Erlangsen et al., 2017). The authors found that in the five years following the death, mental disorder was around twice as common in the group bereaved by suicide compared to those bereaved through other causes. Suicidal behaviours, mortality, and welfare use were also higher in the group who had been bereaved by suicide. Suicide in friends, as well as relatives, seems to infer an increased risk of suicidal behaviours in young adults (Pitman et al., 2016). Suicide bereavement may impact on educational attainment and occupational outcomes (Pitman et al., 2018).

13.3 Differences from other forms of bereavement

Older studies suggested some similarities in morbidity between those bereaved by suicide and those bereaved through other causes. However, those bereaved by suicide receive less emotional support, they often feel stigmatized, and their initial recovery may be slower (Farberow et al., 1992). Factors which can modify bereavement outcomes include: the age of the deceased; the relationship to the deceased; the age, gender, and cultural background of the bereaved; their attitude to the loss; and the quality of their relationship with the deceased. Thus parents of young adults with whom they have had a difficult relationship, and who perceive that they are receiving inadequate support in their grief, may be at particular risk (Grad, 2011).

Suicide may occur in a family which is experiencing multiple psychosocial stressors. There may be a higher prevalence of psychiatric illness. Suicidal behaviour can run in some families, and therefore those bereaved by suicide are an 'at-risk' group, not just because of the mode of death itself but because of possible genetic and environmental vulnerabilities.

There may be differences in the type of help available and accessed after suicide bereavement compared to bereavement by other causes. In a major survey of over three thousand young adults, respondents bereaved by suicide were less likely to receive informal support than people bereaved by other causes of death. They were also more likely to perceive delays in accessing formal or informal help (Pitman et al., 2017c).

13.4 Grief themes

There are certain commonalities to emotional experiences in those who are bereaved following a death by suicide (Clark and Goldney, 1995). An understanding of these themes has come from qualitative studies. In clinical practice it is useful to be aware of them and provide help to address them as appropriate. They are not discrete but overlapping and there is no set chronology for their emergence.

Box 13.1 Grief themes in bereavement through suicide

- Shock, disbelief, horror
- How and why?
- Guilt and blame
- Family reaction
- Stigma, shame, and isolation; a sense of a wasted life
- Suicidal thoughts and fear of another suicide
- Anger
- Aversion versus imitation

Box 13.1 lists some of them, but of course these themes may vary greatly according to the individual and their cultural setting.

13.4.1 Shock

The shock of discovering the deceased may be recurring and long-lasting, with flash backs of finding the body, or experiences of feelings and sensations associated with the event.

13.4.2 Disbelief

Disbelief may be overwhelming and the bereaved person may focus on other explanations for the death. Such convictions may be reinforced by feelings of shame, and it is possible that accounts of the cause of death may be inaccurate.

13.4.3 Horror

The feeling of horror may include the realization of the extreme depth of distress the deceased must have been in. The bereaved person may think repeatedly about the suffering of their loved one and whether the deceased had in fact 'changed his or her mind' but it was too late to act.

13.4.4 How?

The family may wish to know precisely how the person died, including whether drugs or medications were ingested, and the physical and psychiatric effects of those substances. A sensitive interpretation of the post-mortem report or coronial enquiry may be needed.

13.4.5 Why?

This is probably the most common question after bereavement by suicide, and ultimately there is no satisfactory answer. Questions are often asked about what external pressures the deceased was experiencing and why there was a breakdown in communication with regard to seeking help. A suicide note may induce feelings of responsibility and guilt in the bereaved person. Blame from others may also be experienced.

13.4.6 Guilt and blame

Guilt and blame commonly arise from the quest for 'why?'. The bereaved person may feel they contributed to the suicide death and blame themselves for not having prevented it. Mothers and fathers can feel that they were not sufficiently good parents and let their son or daughter down. They may feel that as the closest person to their child, they should have been the ones to see the signs of hopelessness and to have acted as their child's confidante. 'If only ... ' is a common phrase used to describe acts that might have prevented the suicide. Some families feel they did all they could, whereas others, even if they participated fully in the deceased's care, may have unrealistic feelings of remorse. Guilt may also be felt at the sense of relief that those bereaved sometimes experience, particularly those who describe spending many years on 'suicide watch' (Omerov et al., 2013).

13.4.7 Family reaction

For many families, the tragedy of suicide creates upheaval and disaster. This includes families who had previously regarded themselves as functioning normally, and where the suicide death was quite unexpected or 'out of the blue'. For already disadvantaged families with multiple challenges, the suicide death may add to their difficulties. On the other hand, some families who struggle for years with a depressed individual and suicidal behaviours may experience paradoxical relief after a loved one dies. By the time death occurs, the family may have accepted mental illness as the cause of death. They may also be comforted that the deceased is out of distress, even though they regret the means.

13.4.8 Rejection

Suicide is sometimes felt to be a conscious rejection of the family and, in the context of difficult relationships, the bereaved person may interpret the death as a hostile act with no opportunity for redress.

13.4.9 Stigma, shame, and social isolation

The experience of stigma varies between studies and appears to be culturally-based. Even where stigma is absent, feelings of shame may arise due to guilt, blame, rejection, being the subject of gossip, and the association of suicide with mental disorders.

Shame plays an important role in constraining interpersonal relationships and the bereaved person may become socially isolated. There may also be a lack of emotional support for those bereaved through suicide. Community studies indicate a mismatch in knowledge and attitudes between the bereaved and professional or community groups. After a suicide death, the bereaved may have the additional burden of having to discuss the causes and nature of suicide with friends and acquaintances, and even to educate them about how to respond appropriately to someone who has been bereaved. A useful guide for non-professionals about talking to someone bereaved by suicide has recently been published in the UK (https://www.thecalmzone.net/wp-content/uploads/2018/03/Finding_the_Words.pdf).

13.4.10 Lost potential

Remorse at the loss of potential and the missed opportunities for the deceased person and for members of the bereaved family are common themes.

13.4.11 Suicidal thoughts and fear of another suicide death

Suicidal thoughts are common and may be in part a desire to join the deceased, or they can be associated with depression. Fears about further suicide deaths may result in families becoming over-protective. In particular, parents may worry about the risk to younger siblings when they reach the age at which the older child took his/her life. Adolescents may have difficulty dealing with the boundaries between themselves and a role model who died by suicide. Acquaintances may worry about contagion, which may cause them to withdraw support to the bereaved (Pitman et al., 2017c).

13.4.12 Anger

Anger at the deceased may result from the emotional pain experienced, particularly if the bereaved person was blamed in a suicide note, or had offered help to the deceased and had been rejected. When a partner dies by suicide, there may be anger at being cheated out of the relationship or at being left to carry the full burden of the family's responsibilities. Anger may also be expressed towards the healthcare team, God, or the therapist, or towards the press for inaccurate, exaggerated, or sensational reports, and for the loss of privacy at the time of family tragedy (Chapple et al., 2013).

13.4.13 Aversion versus imitation

Data from a recent study of over four hundred young people suggests that for some individuals being bereaved by suicide might make them more averse to ever considering suicide (because of the effect on those left behind), but for others, bereavement might make suicide more an option for them (that is, it increases the cognitive availability) (Pitman et al., 2017a).

13.5 Practical issues and bereavement care

A physician certifying death can sensitively allay initial confusion and provide explanation about such matters as why resuscitation was stopped, or not begun, and the need for official investigation at a time of personal tragedy. It is important to be honest about the presumed cause of death.

Opportunity should be offered to view the body but, if there has been significant injury, the alternative of maintaining vigil over the covered body may be preferred (Chapple et al., 2013). Families may be understandably angry if this opportunity is denied. If a decision is taken not to view the body, discussions should be had with a family member or the funeral director to possibly take photographs of the body in case of future need. These may be useful later to alleviate any thoughts of misidentification ('It wasn't really him that died').

If a public funeral is not held, regrets about not giving adequate tribute to the deceased may arise. In addition, the opportunity for other significant people in the deceased's life (e.g. school friends, work colleagues) to grieve may be denied. If the funeral is private or if there is no funeral at all, the bereaved might also deprive themselves of the support of others.

An explanation of various models of suicide may be helpful in understanding why the deceased took his/her life, and such a no-blame approach may alleviate feelings of guilt, rejection, and shame. Any apparent social stressors or other environmental causes of the suicide death must, of course, be acknowledged. Explanation of the impossibility of prediction of suicide in any individual, even by professionals, may assist in allaying concerns that the bereaved should have prevented the suicide. If there is an internal or external review or inquiry following the death, families should be involved as much as possible.

Counselling may be helpful to assist a bereaved person to deal with unrealistic feelings, particularly guilt, rejection, and those arising from the suicide note. A gentle exploration of feelings, on the basis that the introjection of such feelings contributes to emotional distress, is usually therapeutic, although the timing of such intervention needs careful judgement. Grief counselling may be provided by healthcare or voluntary services (e.g. Cruse in the UK). Having a point of contact with the clinical team may still be helpful even if a referral for voluntary sector services has been made.

Antidepressant or other psychotropic medications may be needed if the bereaved person meets the criteria for psychiatric illness and as an adjunct to the psychological grief work, rather than as a replacement for it. The quest for why the suicide death occurred may become all-consuming. Helping the bereaved person to turn their attention to other grief themes and a focus on 'here and now' issues may be helpful.

In some communities, support groups have developed for those bereaved by suicide (Szumilas and Kutcher, 2011): for example, SOBS in the UK (https://uksobs.org/). They may be helpful to enable people to recognize that their feelings of intense emotional pain are normal and to provide contact with those who have already gone through the experience of suicide bereavement. Other important functions of such groups are those of advocacy within the community and destigmatization. However, these groups are not suitable for everyone and some people prefer an individual approach.

Other psychological interventions may also be of benefit. One of the few controlled trials in suicide bereavement research tested the effectiveness of a family-based grief CBT counselling programme. It found no difference in suicidal ideation or the level of depression between the intervention and control groups 13 months after the suicide death, but the intervention was associated with a reduction in the perception of blame and maladaptive grief reactions (de Groot et al., 2007). A further analysis suggested the intervention might be effective in reducing complicated grief in people who had suicidal ideation (de Groot et al., 2010). Two systematic reviews have concluded that the evidence base is sparse and the methodological quality of published studies was poor, but bereavement groups, writing interventions, and CBT-based treatment might be helpful for subgroups of those bereaved (McDaid et al., 2008; Linde et al., 2017). Whether such programmes will ever demonstrate that they definitively prevent further suicide is difficult because of the statistical power issue—as noted in previous chapters, suicide is thankfully comparatively rare (in terms of absolute frequency) even in high-risk groups. Nevertheless, the potential preventive role is vital (Andriessen and Krysinska, 2012) and 'postvention' is a key component of many suicide prevention strategies.

Internationally, a number of printed and online resources are available for those bereaved by suicide (e.g. Support after Suicide in the UK— http://supportaftersuicide.org.uk/). 'Help is at Hand' in the UK has been positively evaluated and revised extensively with the input of bereaved relatives (Department of Health, 2015). In addition, a number of practice resources have recently been made available to guide the development and evaluation of suicide bereavement services in the UK (Public Health England, 2016).

13.6 The clinician's reaction

The clinician's or therapist's own response to suicide has also received attention, and the effects have been described in a wide range of professionals and volunteers (Hendin et al., 2000; Seguin et al., 2014). There are feelings of personal loss, shock, and sadness, but there may also be relief that intolerable suffering is over and that the stress of professional vigilance has ended. There may be feelings of professional failure, fear for one's reputation, and anger at the deceased for the disruption he/she caused. There may be lasting personal effects such as physical health problems, depression, irrational fears, and deterioration in interpersonal and professional relationships. There may be considerable distress if there is a formal review or inquiry following the death, and such reviews should be carried out sensitively with a 'no-blame' approach.

Other sequelae include depersonalization and distancing from patients and colleagues, or the opposite—over-involvement in the professional role. Absenteeism, fear of anger from the family and of malpractice suits, and even change of career may all occur. Therapists may find themselves in the difficult position of dealing with their own emotions while at the same time being required to provide objective support to the bereaved family, fellow patients of the person who died by suicide, and professional team members.

A recent UK study of general practitioners reported low levels of confidence in dealing with relatives bereaved by suicide, unpreparedness, guilt, and sometimes a reluctance to contact relatives. Deaths had a significant impact on some clinicians but there was little in the way of supervision or support (Foggin et al., 2016).

The evidence base to inform clinicians' or institutions' approaches to dealing with a suicide death is sparse. Recommendations include training to address the personal and professional issues that emerge in the aftermath, a contingency plan and review protocol for the institution, the availability of professional support for the individual therapist, and the involvement of families (Hendin et al., 2000). However, national data from the UK suggest that in a third of cases of patient suicide, the relatives are not contacted by mental health teams with an offer of support or information, and that specific patient-related factors (forensic history, unemployment, drug and alcohol misuse) are associated with a failure to contact the family (Pitman et al., 2017b). Recently there have been a number of training packages developed for professionals (McDonnell et al., 2016).

13.7 Conclusion

People who are bereaved by suicide are themselves at greater risk. Postvention is an important component of suicide prevention strategies internationally. There are important differences in the way the grief is experienced at a personal level. Families bereaved through suicide may be struggling with pre-existing problems, which can complicate the grieving process. Those bereaved can be left with difficult emotions and unanswered questions which are important for professionals and carers to understand so that appropriate bereavement support and intervention can be provided. Figure 13.1 is an infographic summarizing the information in this chapter.

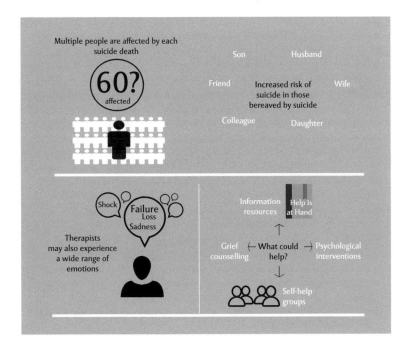

Fig 13.1 Bereavement after suicide.
Courtesy of Dr Sarah Steeg.

REFERENCES

Agerbo, E. (2005). Midlife suicide risk, partner's psychiatric illness, spouse and child bereavement by suicide or other modes of death: a gender specific study. *J Epidemiol Community Health* **59**(5): 407–12.

Andriessen, K. and Krysinska, K. (2012). Essential questions on suicide bereavement and postvention. *Int J Environ Res Public Health* **9**(1): 24–32.

Cerel, J., Brown, M. M., Maple, M., et al. (2019). How many people are exposed to suicide? Not six. *Suicide Life Threat Behav* **49**(2): 529–34.

Chapple, A., Ziebland, S., Simkin, S., and Hawton, K. (2013). How people bereaved by suicide perceive newspaper reporting: qualitative study. *Br J Psychiatry* **203**(3): 228–32.

Clark, S. E. and Goldney, R. D. (1995). Grief reactions and recovery in a support group for people bereaved by suicide. *Crisis* **16**(1): 27–33.

de Groot, M., de Keijser, J., Neeleman, J., Kerkhof, A., Nolen, W., and Burger, H. (2007). Cognitive behaviour therapy to prevent complicated grief among relatives and spouses bereaved by suicide: cluster randomised controlled trial. *BMJ* **334**(7601): 994.

de Groot, M., Neeleman, J., van der Meer, K., and Burger, H. (2010). The effectiveness of family-based cognitive-behavior grief therapy to prevent complicated grief in relatives of suicide victims: the mediating role of suicide ideation. *Suicide Life Threat Behav* **40**(5): 425–37.

Department of Health (2015). *Help is at Hand*. From http://supportaftersuicide.org.uk/wp-content/uploads/2016/09/England-Help-is-at-Hand.pdf

Erlangsen, A., Runeson, B., Bolton, J. M., et al. (2017). Association between spousal suicide and mental, physical, and social health outcomes: a longitudinal and nationwide register-based study. *JAMA Psychiatry* **74**(5): 456–64.

Farberow, N. L., Gallagher-Thompson, D., Gilewski, M., and Thompson, L. (1992). The role of social supports in the bereavement process of surviving spouses of suicide and natural deaths. *Suicide Life Threat Behav* **22**(1): 107–24.

Foggin, E., McDonnell, S., Cordingley, L., Kapur, N., Shaw, J., and Chew-Graham, C. A. (2016). GPs' experiences of dealing with parents bereaved by suicide: a qualitative study. *Br J Gen Pract* **66**(651): e737–46.

Grad, O. (2011). The sequelae of suicide: survivors. In *International Handbook of Suicide Prevention*, R. O'Connor, S. Platt, and J. Gordon (eds). Chichester: John Wiley.

Hendin, H., Lipschitz, A., Maltsberger, J. T., Haas, A. P., and Wynecoop, S. (2000). Therapists' reactions to patients' suicides. *Am J Psychiatry* **157**(12): 2022–7.

Linde, K., Treml, J., Steinig, J., Nagl, M., and Kersting, A. (2017). Grief interventions for people bereaved by suicide: a systematic review. *PLoS One* **12**(6): e0179496.

McDaid, C., Trowman, R., Golder, S., Hawton, K., and Sowden, A. (2008). Interventions for people bereaved through suicide: systematic review. *Br J Psychiatry* **193**(6): 438–43.

McDonnell, S., Kapur, N., Shaw, J., et al. (2016). *Suicide Bereavement Training*. From https://suicidebereavementuk.com/sites/default/files/documents/PABBS_training_competencies.pdf

Omerov, P., Steineck, G., Nyberg, T., Runeson, B., and Nyberg, U. (2013). Psychological morbidity among suicide-bereaved and non-bereaved parents: a nationwide population survey. *BMJ Open* **3**(8): e003108.

Pitman, A., Khrisna Putri, A., De Souza, T., et al. (2018). The impact of suicide bereavement on educational and occupational functioning: a qualitative study of 460 bereaved adults. *Int J Environ Res Public Health* **15**(4): pii: E643. doi: 10.3390/ijerph15040643

Pitman, A., Nesse, H., Morant, N., et al. (2017a). Attitudes to suicide following the suicide of a friend or relative: a qualitative study of the views of 429 young bereaved adults in the UK. *BMC Psychiatry* **17**(1): 400.

Pitman, A., Osborn, D., King, M., and Erlangsen, A. (2014). Effects of suicide bereavement on mental health and suicide risk. *Lancet Psychiatry* **1**(1): 86–94.

Pitman, A. L., Hunt, I. M., McDonnell, S. J., Appleby, A., and Kapur, N. (2017b). Support for relatives bereaved by psychiatric patient suicide: National Confidential Inquiry into Suicide and Homicide findings. *Psychiatric Services* **68**(4): 337–44.

Pitman, A. L., Osborn, D. P. J., Rantell, K., and King, M. B. (2016). Bereavement by suicide as a risk factor for suicide attempt: a cross-sectional national UK-wide study of 3432 young bereaved adults. *BMJ Open* **6**(1): e009948.

Pitman, A. L., Rantell, K., Moran, P. et al. (2017c). Support received after bereavement by suicide and other sudden deaths: a cross-sectional UK study of 3432 young bereaved adults. *BMJ Open* **7**(5): e014487.

Public Health England (2016). *Support After a Suicide: A Guide to Providing Local Services.* From https://www.gov.uk/government/uploads/system/uploads/attachment_data/file/590838/support_after_a_suicide.pdf

Seguin, M., Bordeleau, V., Drouin, M. S., Castelli-Dransart, D. A., and Giasson, F. (2014). Professionals' reactions following a patient's suicide: review and future investigation. *Arch Suicide Res* **18**(4): 340–62.

Szumilas, M. and Kutcher, S. (2011). Post-suicide intervention programs: a systematic review. *Can J Public Health* **102**(1): 18–29.

CHAPTER 14

Frequently asked questions

In this chapter we will aim to answer some common questions about suicide and suicidal behaviour based on the available research evidence. Some of the issues have been touched upon earlier in the book.

14.1 Does asking about suicidal behaviour increase risk?

This question troubles professionals and lay people alike, and may lead to anxiety, avoiding discussion of the issue, or the curtailing of research involving specific questions about suicide, particularly when young people are involved. Clinical experience suggests that the vast majority of those who acknowledge suicidal thoughts or behaviours feel relieved after disclosure.

A comprehensive analysis of the possible risk associated with asking about suicide involved 2,342 students in six high schools in New York State (Gould et al., 2005). All participated in a survey, but half received questions about suicidal behaviour and half did not. A measure of distress was administered to all students at the beginning and end of an initial survey, and at the beginning of a second assessment two days later. The experimental and control groups did not differ on distress levels after the first survey or two days later on measures of mood. Students who had been asked questions about suicide were no more likely to report suicidal ideation compared with the control students. Students who were considered to be at high risk with symptoms of depression, substance use problems, or a past suicide attempt, were neither more suicidal nor more distressed than similar high-risk youth in the control group. Indeed, it was found that those who were depressed and had made a previous suicide attempt were significantly less distressed two days after the initial assessment than high-risk students in the control group—an indication that the enquiry may have been of benefit.

A randomized trial from the UK found that screening for suicidal behaviour did not increase feelings that life was not worth living or suicidal ideation or behaviour (Crawford et al., 2011). A study which examined the effect of qualitative interviews on distress levels found that the majority of participants found the experience cathartic and reported reduced levels of distress after the interview (Biddle et al., 2013). A small number of people reported increased distress, but this was likely to be transient and was outweighed by the wish to contribute to a research project which might help others. Two recent reviews confirm that it is safe to ask about suicide (Dazzi et al., 2014; DeCou and Schumann, 2018). In short, asking about suicide does not increase the risk.

14.2 Is suicide contagious?

The role of the media in propagating suicidal behaviour is well demonstrated and there are media guidelines worldwide which seek to improve the reporting of suicide and minimize the impact on vulnerable individuals (see Chapter 12 for a fuller discussion). Both news media and fictional accounts have been implicated in increasing suicidal behaviour, and mass media is a particular worry because of the number of individuals it reaches. A recent TV series (*13 Reasons Why*) which aired worldwide on the Netflix service attracted huge controversy and led to an increase in suicide-related internet searches (Ayers et al., 2017) and possibly death by suicide (Bridge et al., 2019). However, some have argued that with the increased sophistication of audiences, such mass exposure may not have the impact some fear. Clearly this is an area that needs further research. Media that has worldwide distribution and is not based in any one country presents particular regulatory challenges.

In terms of mechanisms of transmission, some authors distinguish between point clusters and mass clusters (Joiner, 1999). A 'point cluster' may be quite localized, perhaps in an institutional setting like a hospital or a school, and the individuals concerned may have known each other. A 'mass cluster' is generally a media-related phenomenon (sometimes called the 'Werther effect' or, unhelpfully, 'copycat suicide'). One very worrying possibility of sensationalized media coverage of a point cluster is that some kind of mass cluster then becomes superimposed on it. If this is the case, not everyone will be effected equally—young people, individuals who were vulnerable prior to the event, and those who are similar to the victim might be most at risk.

14.3 Can suicide ever be rational?

Are there circumstances in which the decision to take one's own life is rational and understandable? Are there situations in which society and health professionals should respect someone's wishes to die? Legally, in the UK and other countries if someone has capacity (can understand their choices, retain information, weigh everything up, and communicate their decsion) and has no evidence of a mental disorder, then they are free to make treatment choices. From a moral and philosophical viewpoint, personal autonomy might be regarded as paramount and a justification for why people should be able to make their own choices about whether to live or die. Clinically, many mental health professionals would take the pragmatic view that they should try and help and, in an emergency situation, treat first and explore issues around capacity and autonomy later.

Psychological autopsy research suggests up to 90 per cent of people have a psychiatric illness at the time of death by suicide (Cavanagh et al., 2003). Even if levels of formal psychiatric disorder are much less than this, it is clear that sui-cidal behaviour almost always occurs in the context of extreme distress. Suicidal ideas are characterized by ambivalence and changeability. A classic study which interviewed people who survived jumping from bridges in San Francisco showed that all were glad that they had survived (Rosen, 1975). In this context it could be argued that in most cases suicide is not 'rational'. Intervening can buy time and an opportunity for people to change their mind.

Advance decisions or directives in the context of suicidal behaviour—for ex-ample, witnessed specific statements to refuse lifesaving treatment—add even greater complexity and are extremely difficult situations for clinicians to manage (Kapur et al., 2010).

14.3.1 Is euthanasia a special case?

Assisted suicide is different from other forms of suicide because others (commonly physicians) take deliberate action, perhaps to relieve intolerable suffering. Laws vary across the world. In some jurisdictions, euthanasia is per-mitted. In others, for example the UK, it is illegal. Some have argued that on the basis of parity of esteem for psychiatric and physical disorders, euthanasia should be permitted for chronic, severe, unremitting psychological suffering. The Netherlands and Belgium permit assisted dying under these circumstances. Whatever the particular legislative framework, this is an extremely complex area. It may be that societal attitudes to such forms of dying change over time as the population in many Western countries ages. It is clear that assisted dying is different from other forms of suicidal behaviour (Goldney, 2012). For a fuller review of some of the issues for mental health professionals see Sheehan et al. (2017).

14.4 Should people of different ages be managed differently?

The role of mental disorders in the suicidal behaviour of children and ado-lescents is less clear cut than in adults, and more focus needs to be placed on family and interpersonal issues. Furthermore, needs vary across the age range and are not the same for young children and adolescents. Psychiatric illness probably becomes more important during adolescence. Nevertheless, the gen-eral principles of management remain. Suicidal behaviour needs to be taken seriously; a full assessment should be undertaken and management appropriate to the presence or absence of specific disorders needs to be initiated. There should be family involvement, and co-operation with schools and social services may also be required. Antidepressants are probably less effective for young people, and care is needed because of the risk of inducing suicidal thoughts and behaviour early on in treatment. Psychological interventions such as CBT are first-line treatments.

In contrast to young people, suicidal behaviour in those over the age of 55 years is more likely to be associated with diagnosable mental disorders, such as major depression (Lapierre et al., 2011). Suicide attempts are usually of higher suicidal intent and physical lethality, and the ratio of suicide attempts to death by suicide is lower, with attempts being more likely to result in death. The definition of 'late life' varies between settings and changes as the health of populations improves over time, but, in general, physical treatments are more likely to be useful in managing older adults. These treatments include not only psychotropic medication but sometimes alternatives such as electroconvulsive therapy, especially in the context of severe depression. Specific factors which commonly need to be considered in older adults include physical illness, bereavement, and social isolation.

14.5 What does research tell us about 'suicide terrorism'?

'Suicide terrorism' or 'suicide bombing' are commonly used terms to describe similar phenomena, with the terminology often dependent on the context. Clearly these are distinct from what is usually considered to be suicidal behaviour, as the prime motive is the death of others, with the perpetrator's death being incidental. Although most religions prohibit suicide, in some instances such actions have been labelled as 'acts of martyrdom'. They have also been considered as examples of 'altruistic' suicide, but typically altruistic suicide does not involve the death of others.

An early review of suicide terrorism concluded that it had little in common with suicidal behaviour (Townsend, 2007). Similarly, Post et al. referred to the 'normality' and absence of individual psychopathology of suicide bombers (Post et al., 2009). However, one study of perpetrators reported that they had dependent, avoidant, and impulsive personality traits, higher levels of depression, and a greater predisposition to suicidal behaviour than control subjects. The authors concluded that such vulnerable persons would be susceptible to the influence of charismatic leaders (Merari et al., 2009). What seems likely is that psychopathology plays a less important role in 'suicide terrorism' than in suicide more generally.

What mechanisms might be at play in such actions? Social conditioning, cultural sanctioning, a supposed path to spiritual fulfilment, group dynamics, connection with others who have died in this way, and political and military actions based on historical injustices and oppression are all possibilities. In view of these complex motives, and the fact that the primary goal is inflicting death on others, it has also been suggested that the current terminology should be replaced by the term 'homicide bomber' or 'homicide terrorist'. This might have the advantage of not only more accurately describing the action but also indicating that the action is contrary to social and religious conventions (Khan et al., 2010).

Clearly the issues involved in suicide terrorism are wider than mental or population health, and they include individual, societal, and political aspects.

14.6 Are no-harm contracts of value?

Some clinicians treating those who are suicidal devise no-harm contracts as part of a management plan. Typically, these say that the person will not attempt or die by suicide, and that they will adopt different help-seeking behaviour if a crisis arises. However, there is no evidence that they are of value.

The term 'contract' perhaps implies a greater concern for legal obligation, rather than clinical responsibility. It has been suggested that it would be preferable to have a 'commitment to treatment' statement that has elements of manual-based therapy consistent with cognitive behavioural principles (Rudd et al., 2006). However, although such a statement has validity in terms of being more theoretically based, it also has not been subjected to evaluation. 'Safety plans' are a newer development and involve a collaborative process in which the provider and patient list strategies for the patient to use when suicide risk is elevated (Stanley and Brown, 2012). A number of apps offer online safety planning. This is an area of active ongoing research including a number of RCT evaluations.

14.7 Is harm minimization or harm reduction a useful strategy?

One treatment approach that has been used in drug misuse services with a degree of success is harm reduction: for example, providing clean needles or a safe place to use drugs. For some individuals cessation of self-harm may not be a realistic immediate treatment goal. In fact some people report that the release they feel after hurting themselves actually helps to stop them taking their own lives. For these patients, professionals may advocate a 'harm minimization' approach. It has been suggested that harm minimization is about accepting the need to self-harm as a valid method of survival until survival by other means is possible. This does not condone or encourage self-injury but is about facing the reality of self-harm and maximizing safety in the event it occurs (Pembroke, 2007). Some practice-based resources provide information on self-harm as well as outlining distraction techniques, alternatives to self-harm, and damage limitation if self-harm does occur. These approaches are controversial and little researched, and professionals' opinions on their use vary (Gutridge, 2010; James et al., 2017). The NICE guideline on self-harm from the UK (National Collaborating Centre for Mental Health, 2012) suggests that if stopping self-harm is unrealistic in the short term, such strategies might be considered in specialist settings in collaboration with the patient, their carers or significant others, and their clinical team. If such an approach is being adopted, the patient should be advised that there is no safe way to self-poison.

14.8 Has the closure of psychiatric beds contributed to suicide?

In a number of countries there has been a move away from psychiatric in-patient care to more community-focused models of mental health service provision. Some have suggested that this 'deinstitutionalization' may have led to an inadvertent rise in suicide (Goldney, 2003). This was supported by the observation that between 1960 and 1995 mortality rates by suicide rose substantially in six countries in which bed numbers had decreased, whereas only in Japan (which had increased bed numbers during that time) had there been a marginal decline in suicide. Although not specifically addressing deinstitutionalization, the National Confidential Inquiry into Suicide and Homicide in the UK found that suicide was associated with a decrease in the provision of care, including being transferred to a less supervised setting at the last contact, and that remained the case even after controlling for perceived suicide risk (National Confidential Inquiry into Suicide and Homicide by People with Mental Illness, 2001). It also reported that between 1997 and 2003 there could have been as much as a 10 per cent increase in post-discharge suicide, and the possibility that this may have been a transfer of risk from inpatient to outpatient care was raised (Kapur et al., 2006). In addition, there was the later finding that suicide rates were possibly higher in community home-treatment settings than in inpatient wards (Hunt et al., 2014).

On the other hand, a review of post-discharge suicide deaths after deinstitutionalization in Finland, comparing rates from 1985 to 1991 with those from 1995 to 2001, demonstrated a reduction in suicide (Pirkola et al., 2007). It could be argued that the earlier time period was actually after much deinstitutionalization had already occurred, and that the latter period coincided with more intensive suicide prevention measures. In a more detailed analysis, it was reported that the reduction was associated with comprehensive outpatient mental health services (Pirkola et al., 2009). Areas which had well-developed outpatient (versus inpatient) services had a lower suicide rate.

An emphasis on caring for people with mental illness in their own homes rather than admitting them to inpatient wards is well established. However, some service users and clinicians have suggested that the reduction of psychiatric beds may have gone too far. The National Confidential Inquiry in the UK has highlighted safety concerns with 'out of area' admissions, where patients may be admitted hundreds of miles from their homes when there is no local inpatient bed available (National Confidential Inquiry into Suicide and Homicide by People with Mental Illness, 2017). In some areas in the UK and elsewhere, residential crisis centres run by the voluntary or third sector now provide brief respite admissions to fill what they would view as an important gap in statutory services.

Inpatient care remains an important treatment option for people with suicidal thoughts and behaviour, and can sometimes be lifesaving (Large and Kapur, 2018). What is also clear is that community treatment services for people with suicidal thoughts and behaviours need themselves to be safe, evidence-based, well-staffed, and appropriately resourced.

14.9 Are individual inquiries about suicide useful?

This question relates to inquiries about individual suicide deaths which may occur during the course of clinical practice. Naturally, many will be subject to a coroner's hearing (or similar investigation) but some will also be investigated by local hospital or community boards.

When a suicide death occurs, the antecedents often seem clear in retrospect, and investigating teams sometimes conclude that various interventions should or should not have been implemented , and that they would have influenced the outcome. This often leads to blame—self-blame and also blame at the level of individual clinicians or clinical teams—and as a consequence inquiries may be perceived as threatening (Pridmore et al., 2006).

In conducting an inquiry into suicide, the first and often most pressing question from the point of view of service managers and those bereaved by suicide is whether or not the death could have been prevented. This is often an impossible question to answer. The second and equally important question is whether or not management practices were within the realms of good clinical care. That is, where an objective reviewer can be reassured that there was appropriate management and that the suicide death was an unexpected outcome. On the other hand, if clinical practice was found wanting, this must be highlighted, albeit with the caveat that even if things had been done differently there is no guarantee that the suicide death would have been prevented.

Those entrusted with the important and time-consuming duty of conducting or participating in inquiries after suicide should be aware that patient suicide is particularly distressing. Inappropriately harsh criticisms can be destructive for both individual clinicians and teams, particularly when there are systemic organizational shortcomings which have placed high demands on staff. For an inquiry to be useful, the focus needs to be on identifying areas that can be improved, rather than apportioning blame. Guidance on learning from adverse incidents has been published for health services overall and and mental health services specifically. . Some of the key principles include: prioritizing the most serious cases that require full investigation; involving the patient and their families; supporting and engaging staff; using skilled analysis to identify causes; and adopting human-factor approaches to developing solutions (Care Quality Commission, 2016; Royal College of Psychiatrists, 2018).

The overall purpose of any investigation should be seen as avoiding future harm. Investigations should have clear terms of reference, involve families, be transparent and independent, and be carried out by staff with appropriate training and time. Information sharing between different agencies is an important principle. Reports and recommendations should be succinct and clear. Finally, any actions should balance learning with accountability.

REFERENCES

Ayers, J. W., Althouse, B. M., Leas, E. C., Dredze, M., and Allem, J. P. (2017). Internet searches for suicide following the release of *13 Reasons Why*. *JAMA Intern Med* **177**(10): 1527–9.

Biddle, L., Cooper, J., Owen-Smith, A., et al. (2013). Qualitative interviewing with vulnerable populations: individuals' experiences of participating in suicide and self-harm based research. *J Affect Disord* **145**(3): 356–62.

Bridge, J. A., Greenhouse, J. B., Ruch, D., et al. (2019). Association between the release of Netflix's '13 Reasons Why' and suicide rates in the United States: an interrupted times series analysis. *J Am Acad Child Adolesc Psychiatry*. https://doi.org/10.1016/j.jaac.2019.04.020

Care Quality Commission (2016). *Briefing: Learning from Serious Incidents in NHS Acute Hospitals*. From https://www.cqc.org.uk/publications/themed-work/briefing-learning-serious-incidents-nhs-acute-hospitals

Cavanagh, J. T., Carson, A. J., Sharpe, M., and Lawrie, S. M. (2003). Psychological autopsy studies of suicide: a systematic review. *Psychol Med* **33**(3): 395–405.

Crawford, M. J., Thana, L., Methuen, C., et al. (2011). Impact of screening for risk of suicide: randomised controlled trial. *Br J Psychiatry* **198**(5): 379–84.

Dazzi, T., Gribble, R., Wessely, S., and Fear, N. T. (2014). Does asking about suicide and related behaviours induce suicidal ideation? What is the evidence? *Psychol Med* **44**(16): 3361–3.

DeCou, C. R. and Schumann, M. E. (2018). On the iatrogenic risk of assessing suicidality: a meta-analysis. *Suicide Life Threat Behav* **48**(5): 531–43.

Goldney, R. D. (2003). Deinstitutionalization and suicide. *Crisis* **24**(1): 39–40.

Goldney, R. D. (2012). Neither euthanasia nor suicide, but rather assisted death. *Aust N Z J Psychiatry* **46**(3): 185–7.

Gould, M. S., Marrocco, F. A., Kleinman, M., et al. (2005). Evaluating iatrogenic risk of youth suicide screening programs: a randomized controlled trial. *JAMA* **293**(13): 1635–43.

Gutridge, K. (2010). Safer self-injury or assisted self-harm? *Theor Med Bioeth* **31**(1): 79–92.

Hunt, I. M., Rahman, M. S., While, D., et al. (2014). Safety of patients under the care of crisis resolution home treatment services in England: a retrospective analysis of suicide trends from 2003 to 2011. *Lancet Psychiatry* **1**(2): 135–41.

James, K., Samuels, I., Moran, P., and Stewart, D. (2017). Harm reduction as a strategy for supporting people who self-harm on mental health wards: the views and experiences of practitioners. *J Affect Disord* **214**: 67–73.

Joiner, T. E. (1999). The clustering and contagion of suicide. *Curr Dir Psychol Sci* **8**(3): 89–92.

Kapur, N., Clements, C., Bateman, N., et al. (2010). Advance directives and suicidal behaviour. *BMJ* **341**: c4557.

Kapur, N., Hunt, I. M., Webb, R., et al. (2006). Suicide in psychiatric in-patients in England, 1997 to 2003. *Psychol Med* **36**(10): 1485–92.

Khan, M. M., Goldney, R., and Hassan, R. (2010). Homicide bombers: life as a weapon. *Asian J Soc Sci* **38**(3): 481–4.

Lapierre, S., Erlangsen, A., Waern, M., et al. (2011). A systematic review of elderly suicide prevention programs. *Crisis* **32**(2): 88–98.

Large, M. M. and Kapur, N. (2018). Psychiatric hospitalisation and the risk of suicide. *Br J Psychiatry* **212**(5): 269–73.

Merari, A., Diamant, I., Bibi, A., Broshi, Y., and Zakin, G. (2009). Personality characteristics of 'self martyrs'/ 'suicide bombers' and organizers of suicide attacks. *Terror Pol Viol* **22**(1): 87–101.

National Collaborating Centre for Mental Health (2012). *Self-Harm: Longer-Term Management.* Leicester: British Psychological Society.

National Confidential Inquiry into Suicide and Homicide by People with Mental Illness (2001). *Safety First: Five-Year Report of the National Confidential Inquiry into Suicide and Homicide by People with Mental Illness.* London: Department of Health Publications.

National Confidential Inquiry into Suicide and Homicide by People with Mental Illness (2017). *Annual Report: England, Northern Ireland, Scotland and Wales.* From http:// documents.manchester.ac.uk/display.aspx?DocID=37560

Pembroke, L. (2007). Harm-minimisation: limiting the damage of self-injury. In *Beyond Fear and Control: Working with Young People Who Self-Harm*, H. Spandler and S. Warner (eds). Ross-on-Wye: PCCS Books.

Pirkola, S., Sohlman, B., Heila, H., and Wahlbeck, V. (2007). Reductions in postdischarge suicide after deinstitutionalization and decentralization: a nationwide register study in Finland. *Psychiatr Serv* **58**(2): 221–6.

Pirkola, S., Sund, R., Sailas, E., and Wahlbeck, K. (2009). Community mental-health services and suicide rate in Finland: a nationwide small-area analysis. *Lancet* **373**(9658): 147–53.

Post, J. M., Ali, F., Henderson, S. W., Shanfield, S., Victoroff, J., and Weine, S. (2009). The psychology of suicide terrorism. *Psychiatry* **72**(1): 13–31.

Pridmore, S., Ahmadi, J., and Evenhuis, M. (2006). Suicide for scrutinizers. *Australas Psychiatry* **14**(4): 359–64.

Rosen, D. H. (1975). Suicide survivors. A follow-up study of persons who survived jumping from the Golden Gate and San Francisco-Oakland Bay Bridges. *West J Med* **122**(4): 289–94.

Royal College of Psychiatrists (2018). *Principles for Full Investigation of Serious Incidents Involving Patients under the Care of Mental Health and Intellectual Disability Provider Organisations.* From https://www.rcpsych.ac.uk/usefulresources/publications/ collegereports/op/op104.aspx

Rudd, M. D., Mandrusiak, M., and Joiner Jr., T. E. (2006). The case against no-suicide contracts: the commitment to treatment statement as a practice alternative. *J Clin Psychol* **62**(2): 243–51.

Sheehan, K., Gaind, K. S., and Downar, J. (2017). Medical assistance in dying: special issues for patients with mental illness. *Curr Opin Psychiatry* **30**(1): 26–30.

Stanley, B. and Brown, G. K. (2012). Safety planning intervention: a brief intervention to mitigate suicide risk. *Cogn Behav Pract* **19**(2): 256–64.

Townsend, E. (2007). Suicide terrorists: are they suicidal? *Suicide Life Threat Behav* **37**(1): 35–49.

CHAPTER 15

Conclusion

KEY POINTS

- No single approach is suitable for all.
- Effective strategies are available which can be tailored to specific situations or individuals.
- We should not neglect the management of mental health problems in people who present with suicidal thoughts or behaviours.
- It is sometimes argued that the evidence base is weak, but suicide prevention research of the highest quality is being produced at an increasing rate.
- Future work might harness the power of large health and population datasets, develop and implement effective interventions, make use of new technology, involve service users and relatives, and focus on low- and middle-income countries where most deaths occur.
- The challenges of ageing populations and the provision of health services under economically constrained circumstances will also need to be addressed.
- By using some of the strategies that have been developed internationally there is every reason to be optimistic that rates of suicide worldwide can be reduced.

15.1 The knowledge base

The suggestion that there is little evidence for the effectiveness of suicide prevention measures is less than convincing. Of course, it is unrealistic to expect a single approach to suit everyone (Pitman, 2007), but there are a number of interventions which appear to work and which can be adapted for different countries and different clinical populations (Goldney, 2005; Mann et al., 2005; Zalsman et al., 2016).

The causes of suicide are varied and complex. Broad societal influences such as socioeconomic factors and social integration are associated with rates of suicide. Access to high-lethality methods contributes to suicide, as does sensationalized or prominent media reporting. Birth cohort studies have investigated the interrelationship between early developmental risk factors and subsequent suicidal behaviour. Twin studies have confirmed the importance of both inherited and environmental factors. There have been investigations of the biology of suicidal behaviour; and detailed clinical and non-clinical studies have highlighted the importance of individual psychological factors (e.g. perceived interpersonal rejection) in precipitating the final act.

Research which has tried to place risk factors in perspective (e.g. studies which calculate the population-attributable risk) has shown that mental health problems are very important at an individual level, especially in higher-income countries. These are potentially modifiable factors which can be addressed by the clinician or individual themselves rather than requiring legislative or societal action. It is acknowledged that the predominantly clinical approach may be less appropriate in lower-income countries (Phillips, 2010). However, even in such settings the clinician's imperative is to ensure that any underlying clinical disorders are treated.

It is important to reflect on research that has demonstrated that standard treatments do not appear to have been used with a significant proportion of those who die by suicide (Marzuk et al., 1995). That is consistent with findings from the UK and Australia that perhaps 20 per cent of suicide deaths in association with hospitalization may have been preventable, but for poor staff–patient relationships, inadequate assessment and management of depression and other disorders, and poor continuity of care, particularly in the transition period between hospitalization and the community (Burgess et al., 2000; National Confidential Inquiry into Suicide and Homicide by People with Mental Illness, 2001). Equally for non-fatal suicidal behaviour, work suggests that only 60 per cent of people receive an adequate assessment if they present to hospital services after having harmed themselves (Cooper et al., 2013). These gaps in service provision clearly need to be addressed.

There are formidable methodological challenges when investigating suicide within health services, but clinical interventions are crucial components of suicide prevention (Tondo et al., 2006). There are reports of the benefits of policy recommendations in enhancing mental health service safety and reducing suicide (While et al., 2012) and attempted suicide (Gunnell et al., 2012). Indeed, such findings have led to the recommendation that such policy initiatives should be adopted internationally (Appleby, 2012). Perhaps at least as important as the policy initiatives themselves is the organizational context in which changes are made (Kapur et al., 2016). Service changes will always have more of an impact in well-run, stable health services.

15.2 Future priorities for practice, policy, and research

Population-based measures can help to reduce suicide. Researchers, clinicians, patients, and families all have a role to play in influencing decision makers and those who plan health and social care policy. Clinical services are also important. Not all professionals will manage people with suicidal thoughts or behaviours. However, they should all possess the clinical skills to make a general assessment and management plan, perhaps with a view to referral to a colleague or service with specific interest. These generic skills should include an assessment of psychosocial context as well as psychiatric illness.

Future opportunities for research include harnessing the power of linked large datasets—'big data'—to improve our aetiological understanding of suicide. But we also need to move on from pure risk-factor research to better characterize what works in the real world. We need to develop, test, and implement effective pharmacological, psychological, social, and societal interventions on a large scale (National Action Alliance for Suicide Prevention: Research Prioritization Task Force, 2014). Randomized controlled trials are in one sense a gold standard but may not be feasible given the population incidence of suicide.

We should use a variety of innovative research methods. Intervening in the digital space and making use of new technologies may help us to reach more people than ever before. Meaningful involvement of patients and their families, as well as those bereaved by suicide, will reap dividends. Much of the work to date has been carried out in Western settings—not in low- and middle-income countries where most suicide deaths occur. The WHO has recommended a focus on developing high-quality suicide prevention strategies and robust data collection internationally (WHO, 2014). There will be challenges in the worldwide effort to prevent suicide. For example, how should suicide prevention efforts respond to the rapidly ageing populations in many countries? How should we address the difficulty of providing equitable health services under economically constrained circumstances?

Decades of research into suicide prevention has provided an evidence base, and one that is growing all the time. Yes, the evidence may be imperfect, but that should not be used as an excuse for inaction. Addressing the implementation gap—that is, the lack of routine availability of interventions we know to be effective—is an immediate priority. In the past there may have been a sense of pessimism about our capacity to prevent suicidal behaviour, but this is no longer warranted. By using knowledge gained from two centuries of suicide prevention research, and by putting it into practice, there is every reason to believe that the rate of suicide worldwide can be reduced.

REFERENCES

Appleby, L. (2012). Suicide prevention: the evidence on safer clinical care is now good and should be adopted internationally. *Int Psychiatry* 9: 27–9.

Burgess, P., Pirkis, J., Morton, J., and Croke, E. (2000). Lessons from a comprehensive clinical audit of users of psychiatric services who committed suicide. *Psychiatr Serv* 51(12): 1555–60.

Cooper, J., Steeg, S., Bennewith, O., et al. (2013). Are hospital services for self-harm getting better? An observational study examining management, service provision and temporal trends in England. *BMJ Open* 3(11): e003444.

Goldney, R. D. (2005). Suicide prevention: a pragmatic review of recent studies. *Crisis* 26(3): 128–40.

Gunnell, D., Metcalfe, C., While, D., et al. (2012). Impact of national policy initiatives on fatal and non-fatal self-harm after psychiatric hospital discharge: time series analysis. *Br J Psychiatry* **201**(3): 233–8.

Kapur, N., Ibrahim, S., While, D., et al. (2016). Mental health service changes, organisational factors, and patient suicide in England in 1997–2012: a before-and-after study. *Lancet Psychiatry* **3**(6): 526–34.

Mann, J. J., Apter, A., Bertolote, J., et al. (2005). Suicide prevention strategies: a systematic review. *JAMA* **294**(16): 2064–74.

Marzuk, P. M., Tardiff, K., Leon, A. C., et al. (1995). Use of prescription psychotropic drugs among suicide victims in New York City. *Am J Psychiatry* **152**(10): 1520–2.

National Action Alliance for Suicide Prevention: Research Prioritization Task Force (2014). *A prioritized research agenda for suicide prevention: an action plan to save lives.* From https://theactionalliance.org/sites/default/files/agenda.pdf

National Confidential Inquiry into Suicide and Homicide by People with Mental Illness (2001). *Safety First: Five-Year Report of the National Confidential Inquiry into Suicide and Homicide by People with Mental Illness.* London: Department of Health Publications.

Phillips, M. R. (2010). Rethinking the role of mental illness in suicide. *Am J Psychiatry* **167**(7): 731–3.

Pitman, A. (2007). Policy on the prevention of suicidal behaviour; one treatment for all may be an unrealistic expectation. *J R Soc Med* **100**(10): 461–4.

Tondo, L., Albert, M. J., and Baldessarini, R. J. (2006). Suicide rates in relation to health care access in the United States: an ecological study. *J Clin Psychiatry* **67**(4): 517–23.

While, D., Bickley, H., Roscoe, A., et al. (2012). Implementation of mental health service recommendations in England and Wales and suicide rates, 1997–2006: a cross-sectional and before-and-after observational study. *Lancet* **379**(9820): 1005–12.

World Health Organization (2014). *Preventing Suicide: A Global Imperative 2014.* From http://www.who.int/mental_health/suicide-prevention/world_report_2014/en/

Zalsman, G., Hawton, K., Wasserman, D., et al. (2016). Suicide prevention strategies revisited: 10-year systematic review. *Lancet Psychiatry* **3**(7): 646–59.

CHAPTER 15

CHAPTER 16

Clinical examples

> **KEY POINTS**
>
> - All those who present with suicidal thought and behaviours warrant full assessment.
> - The treatment offered depends on the presence and nature of any psychiatric and physical illnesses identified, as well as wider patient needs.
> - Older persons may have more prominent mental disorders.
> - Some form of follow-up should be offered whenever possible.

16.1 Introduction

These three case histories illustrate common situations encountered by clinicians who have responsibility for patients presenting with suicidal thoughts or behaviours. They are brief. Usually a much more detailed personal history and description of the suicidal behaviour is taken. However, insofar as any person's life experience is similar to another, they depict a young person with interpersonal issues, a person with a long history of behaviours that might fit the criteria for borderline personality disorder, and a man in mid-life with a severe psychiatric illness.

16.2 Amanda

Amanda was an 18-year-old university student who took an overdose of 15 benzodiazepine tablets (belonging to her mother) after her boyfriend had ended their relationship. Things had been difficult for about six months. On a previous occasion when she had threatened self-harm, her boyfriend had rallied around and had been supportive. However, on this occasion he had emphasized that their break-up was final. She took the tablets in her bedroom, knowing that her mother would come to wake her in the morning. Her mother found her to be barely rousable. After assessment in a general hospital emergency department, where she reported not being able to remember what had happened, she was admitted to a short-stay psychiatric ward.

In her family history she was the youngest, by six years, of three children, and her mother had been ambivalent about the pregnancy. However, Amanda remembered being her father's favourite. She had felt particularly distressed when her parents separated when she was aged seven. She saw her father only infrequently after that. Her mother had had several difficult relationships, including one with a man who attempted to sexually assault Amanda. That had led to an estrangement from her mother, who felt that Amanda may have provoked the episode.

Following admission, Amanda indicated that she had not cared whether she had lived or died. She thought that the 15 tablets she had taken would probably not have killed her, but would have allowed her to block out any feelings. Initially, she was tearful and depressed. The admitting team made a provisional diagnosis of an adjustment disorder.

Within 48 hours (during which time there had been a joint interview with her and her mother, and contact from her father) she had improved significantly and was discharged. A home visit by a social worker, after three days, confirmed that Amanda was coping well, but she was embarrassed, being unable to understand why she had risked her life. There was further follow-up two weeks later, when she was introspective and wished to explore her feelings about her parents. Three sessions of interpersonal therapy were undertaken. She found these helpful and was able to see a connection between her sensitivity to rejection and how she had felt as a child in relation to her parents and her mother's partners. Although there was some fluctuation in her mood, she decided to not pursue further therapy, but agreed to re-establish contact if the need arose.

This vignette illustrates the interpersonal nature of suicidal behaviour and the importance of taking a longitudinal history to identify potential sources of early rejection, which can be re-experienced in the context of current relationships. This is particularly so when role models also have unsatisfactory relationships. It also illustrates the potential dangerousness of ambivalence—that is, people not caring whether they live or die. Small amounts of medication, particularly if taken with alcohol, can result in death in vulnerable individuals, even though suicidal intent may not appear to be great. The NICE self-harm guidelines from the UK make it clear that self-poisoning is never 'safe'.

16.3 Sally

Sally was a 33-year-old woman who presented to an emergency department the morning after having taken 20 olanzapine tablets. She said she had taken them in her car in a country park the night before, expecting to die. She was surprised when she woke up, and thought she should go to hospital. She had argued with her partner. She saw no real hope for the future. The olanzapine she took had been prescribed for her some months previously but she said it had not really helped, as it made her feel 'spaced out'.

She had a history of self-harm episodes with serious intent on three previous occasions, the first when aged 16. In addition, there was an extensive history of less medically serious self-harm, with her cutting and burning her arms and thighs. She had been treated by psychiatrists, psychologists, and social workers in the past, but she had always broken off therapy. She felt that therapists did not really care about her.

Her personal life was challenging. She had been in a number of relationships and had had three terminations of pregnancy. Currently, she was in an abusive relationship with a younger man who had recently been the subject of a court order for violence. She was the younger of non-identical twins and also had two younger siblings. Her younger siblings had different fathers. Her mother had a history of multiple overdoses and hospitalizations, and few long-term relationships. Sally had been on unemployment and sickness benefits for six years.

Examining her case notes, it appeared that although she had been assessed and treated by a number of different practitioners, no long-term therapeutic relationship had ever been established. Sally had never received formal psychotherapy. She was considered by the assessing clinical team to have a borderline personality disorder and was offered a place in a dialectical behaviour therapy (DBT) programme. However, she declined. She said she felt that nobody could help her, and she discharged herself from the emergency department. Although she had declined follow-up, she had consented to being contacted by telephone. Contact was made with her three days and then two weeks after she had left the emergency department. Two months later she re-presented with superficial lacerations of her left forearm in the context of further violence from her partner. After accepting treatment for her lacerations, she also accepted entry into a DBT programme.

Over a period of 12 months her mood gradually improved. There was no further self-harm, although she attended an emergency department on one occasion in distress. She also had phone contact with her therapist. She still felt unable to work , but she had ended her abusive relationship and was living independently. During therapy she sometimes found it difficult to see the link between her thoughts and behaviours. She did see some connection between her behaviour and that of her family, particularly her mother.

This vignette illustrates the longitudinal history of someone with longstanding interpersonal difficulties who was diagnosed as having borderline personality disorder by clinical services. It also highlights the fact that sometimes therapists need to persevere. In the clinical situation it may be that a person experiences a number of years of disrupted life and difficult personal relationships before they are willing to engage in therapy.

16.4 Malcolm

Malcolm was a 55-year-old businessman who was found in a hotel room by a cleaner. He was deeply unconscious and a suicide note was by his bed. Two empty bottles of sleeping tablets were also found. He had written an apology to his wife for the nature of his death. He wrote that his business life had been a failure and that he had been a 'pretender' in all his activities, work and social. It subsequently emerged that he had searched the internet for methods of suicide and had purchased the tablets from an online source. After resuscitation in an intensive care unit he appeared to be profoundly depressed, with psychomotor retardation and feelings of guilt. Initially, he was considered to have a severe depressive episode.

His wife expressed considerable concern about her husband. He had left for work the day before, appearing to be quite distressed, and then did not return home. She had informed the police. She said that his work colleagues had indicated that his performance had deteriorated in the last few months. Previously he had been highly successful in his career.

His wife noted that her husband's father had died by suicide in his mid-fifties some 30 years before, and her husband had confided in her that he feared that he would not live beyond his father's age. His wife also reported that at times, over the years, her husband had been quite overactive, and this had probably led to him being particularly successful in his sales field. She also said that she was aware that he had attended university for two years, before she met him, but that he had dropped out after becoming withdrawn and introspective.

The assessing team felt that Malcolm's longitudinal history was suggestive of a bipolar affective disorder, with the first depressive episode being in his early twenties, followed by episodes of subclinical overactivity or hypomania. However, the presenting problem was that of a profound depression, which, after a complete history was collated, was felt to be the depressed phase of a bipolar disorder.

Malcolm had very prominent depressive and guilt-ridden ruminations on admission to the psychiatric inpatient unit which persisted over two weeks, during which time he threatened to abscond in order to kill himself. He was detained on a compulsory basis under the local Mental Health Act. He stopped eating and drinking and became almost mute. The admitting team decided on a course of electroconvulsive therapy and six unilateral treatments were undertaken with a good response. Malcolm was discharged a week later. At outpatient follow-up after two months, he became overactive and, after discussion about potential side effects, lithium was introduced. Over a period of six weeks Malcolm's mood stabilized, and at two-year follow-up he was coping well. There had been no recurrence of suicidal ideation. He was experiencing no side effects from the lithium and blood levels were satisfactory. In view of how settled he felt, he agreed to remain on the lithium indefinitely.

This vignette illustrates the potential for bipolar disorders to result in intense suicidal thoughts and behaviour in the depressed phase. It also illustrates the importance of a family and longitudinal history, including from an independent informant. Often in the clinical setting, a diagnosis of bipolar disorder can only be made with confidence after such history-taking. Lithium is a well-established treatment for those with bipolar disorder, particular if suicidal ideation is expressed. The family history of suicide, longitudinal history of mood swings, and lethality of his suicide attempt may be factors in favour of recommending indefinite use of lithium, subject to the usual monitoring requirements.

CHAPTER 17

Useful links

With the increasing recognition of suicide as a major health and social issue, many suicide prevention organizations have been established locally, nationally, and internationally. A number of these are referred to in this chapter, but the list is indicative rather than exhaustive. We have not included individual research centres, of which there are many.

16.1 International organizations

International Association for Suicide Prevention (IASP)

The IASP was founded in Vienna in 1960 and is a non-profit organization with official affiliation to the World Health Organization. Members from over 50 countries include researchers, clinicians, volunteers, and other professionals who share their knowledge and collaborate on suicide prevention worldwide. International congresses are held every two years and regional conferences are also co-sponsored. Further information is available at: https://www.iasp.info/

International Academy of Suicide Research (IASR)

The IASR was established in 1990 as a forum to promote and disseminate research into suicidal behaviours. Further information is available at: https://suicide-research.org

The Samaritans

The Samaritans was established in 1953 in England and aims to ensure that fewer people die by suicide. It provides telephone and online emotional support, and has over two hundred branches in the UK and Ireland, but is also represented internationally. The Samaritans has received 68 million contacts since 1984. Further information is available at: www.samaritans.org

Befrienders Worldwide

Befrienders Worldwide evolved from the Samaritans, and until 2003 it was known as Befrienders International. It was launched as an independent charity in 2012 and runs nearly 350 emotional support centres in 32 countries, helping an estimated seven million people per year. Further information is available at: www.befrienders.org

Lifeline International

Lifeline International was established in 1963 in Australia, and provides services in 15 countries, predominantly in the southern hemisphere. Further information is available at: https://www.lifeline.org.au

International Federation of Telephone Emergency Services (IFOTES)

IFOTES was founded in 1967 and is now represented in 25 countries, predominantly in Europe. Further information is available at: www.ifotes.org

World Health Organization

The WHO pages are a very useful resource on the prevention of suicide and suicidal behaviour globally. They can be found at: http://www.who.int/mental_health/suicide-prevention/en/

16.2 National suicide prevention organizations and initiatives

Australia: Suicide Prevention Australia

Details available at: http://suicidepreventionaust.org/

Canada: Canadian Association for Suicide Prevention

Details available at: www.suicideprevention.ca/

Germany: German Association for Suicide Prevention

Details available at: http://www.suizidprophylaxe.de/

Ireland: Irish Association of Suicidology

Details available at: www.ias.ie/

New Zealand: Suicide Prevention Information New Zealand (SPINZ)

Details available at: www.spinz.org.nz

The Netherlands

Details available at: https://www.113.nl/english

Nordic countries: Nordic Consortium on Suicide Prevention (NSP)

Details available at: http://nordicsuicideprevention.org/

CHAPTER 17

Taiwan: Taiwanese Society of Suicidology

Details available at: http://tspc.tw/tspc/portal/index/

Thailand: The Suicide Prevention of Thailand Project

Details available at: www.suicidethai.com

United States of America: American Association of Suicidology

Details available at: www.suicidology.org

United States of America: American Foundation for Suicide Prevention

Details available at: http://www.afsp.org/

United Kingdom

Statistics

https://www.ons.gov.uk/
https://fingertips.phe.org.uk/profile-group/mental-health/profile/suicide

Policy

https://www.gov.uk/government/collections/suicide-prevention-resources-and-guidance
http://www.chooselife.net/
http://www.wales.nhs.uk/sitesplus/888/page/65108
https://www.health-ni.gov.uk/articles/suicide-prevention

Third and voluntary sector

http://www.nspa.org.uk/

16.3 Other organizations

Many other volunteer organizations have been established, including Sneha in Tamil Nadu (available at: www.snehaindia.org), Maithri in Kerala, India (available at: http://maithrikochin.org/home.htm), Sumithrayo in Sri Lanka (available at: www.srilankasumithrayo.org/), and Inochi no Denwa in Japan (available at: http://www.inochinodenwa.org).

Index

Tables, figures, and boxes are indicated by an italic *t*, *f*, and *b* following the page/paragraph number

For the benefit of digital users, indexed terms that span two pages (e.g., 52–53) may, on occasion, appear on only one of those pages.